Intimacy, Sex and Relationship Challenges Laid Bare Across the Lifespan

This accessible book uses case studies to explore issues around intimacy, sexual function and sexual development over the lifespan, introducing applied principles and practices when working with sexuality-related issues.

Introducing an easy-to-use 'Reflect and Respond' model as a framework for interactions, this book discusses a broad selection of topics and life stages, including hidden loss, gender identity, disability, early years experiences and older age. Exposing anonymised real-life experiences of intimacy, sexual function and sexual development from birth to end of life, the book develops the reader's insight into sexual wellbeing and confidence in communicating about it. The experiential learning and research-based content in readable style will educate and inspire readers with an interest in sexual wellbeing and how this impacts on physical and mental health.

Demonstrating how being open to talk about sex and intimacy can change lives, this guide is suitable for a wide range of health and social care professionals, including nurses, doctors, occupational therapists, social workers, psychologists and counsellors.

Judy Benns was a registered nurse for 42 years and spent 30 years specialising in sexual health, including HIV, contraception and psychosexual therapy. Prior to retiring, she worked as a clinical nurse manager for a nurse-led contraception and sexual health service. Judy keeps updated with research and developments in contraception and sexual health provision, in particular for young people.

Sue Burridge qualified as a direct entry midwife when she also facilitated a clinic for women experiencing vaginismus. She trained in psychosexual therapy and practice and is a member of the College of Sex and Relationship Therapists (COSRT). More recently, Sue has utilised her experience to progress to leading on the commissioning of contraception and sexual health service provision.

Jean Penman is a former nurse specialist and holds a senior accreditation with the British Association for Counselling & Psychotherapy, specialising in psychosexual counselling. She was awarded a Professional Doctorate for her specialist research interest, 'Engaging with medically unexplained physical symptoms in healthcare', at the Institute of Health & Social Care, University of Bedfordshire, England in 2016.

11 Mid-life   127

12 Older age   144

13 Supervision   150

    Epilogue   161
    Index   163

Contents

List of illustrations	vii
List of case studies	viii
Preface	xiii
List of abbreviations and clarification of terms	xvi
Introduction	1
1 Experiences in early years	20
2 Reproductive years	36
3 Losses in reproductive years	47
4 Unexpected outcomes and sexual development	57
5 Mental health	65
6 Gender identity, sexuality and difference in sexual desire	73
7 Sexual health	94
8 Women's health	108
9 Marriage and civil partnership	114
10 Hidden loss	120

First published 2021
by Routledge
2 Park Square, Milton Park, Abingdon, Oxon OX14 4RN

and by Routledge
52 Vanderbilt Avenue, New York, NY 10017

Routledge is an imprint of the Taylor & Francis Group, an informa business

© 2021 Judy Benns, Sue Burridge and Jean Penman

The rights of Judy Benns, Sue Burridge and Jean Penman to be identified as authors of this work has been asserted by them in accordance with sections 77 and 78 of the Copyright, Designs and Patents Act 1988.

All rights reserved. No part of this book may be reprinted or reproduced or utilised in any form or by any electronic, mechanical, or other means, now known or hereafter invented, including photocopying and recording, or in any information storage or retrieval system, without permission in writing from the publishers.

Trademark notice: Product or corporate names may be trademarks or registered trademarks, and are used only for identification and explanation without intent to infringe.

British Library Cataloguing-in-Publication Data
A catalogue record for this book is available from the British Library

Library of Congress Cataloging-in-Publication Data
A catalog record has been requested for this book

ISBN: 978-0-367-71325-6 (hbk)
ISBN: 978-0-367-71321-8 (pbk)
ISBN: 978-1-003-15031-2 (ebk)

Typeset in Bembo
by Deanta Global Publishing Services, Chennai, India

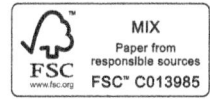 Printed in the United Kingdom
by Henry Ling Limited

Intimacy, Sex and Relationship Challenges Laid Bare Across the Lifespan

Applied Principles and Practice for Health Professionals

Judy Benns, Sue Burridge and Jean Penman

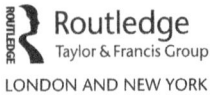

LONDON AND NEW YORK

Illustrations

Figures

0.1	The expert and the patient. Source: Penman, 1998	3
0.2	The comforter. Source: Penman, 1998	4
0.3	The therapeutic space developed through the practitioner–patient relationship. Source: Penman, 1998	6
0.4	Finding the heart of the matter: underpinning factors which may be found when talking to people with sexual dysfunction or sexual dissatisfaction	8
0.5	Therapy process: themes discovered during an intervention for reducing persistent sexual symptoms. Source: Penman, 2015	9
0.6	Examples of physical and emotional motivations for sex and intimacy	12
1.1	The cycle of unresolved persistent physical symptoms (uPPS). Source: Penman, 2015	25

Table

0.1	Reflect and Respond model process template: recording learning and practice development	7

Case studies

Chapter	Section	Title of case study	Condition
Experiences in early years	Influences on sexual development	Celine: Am I normal?	No feeling during sex
	Disruption to sexual development	Amanda's disconnection	Loss of sexual desire
		Ben's buried loss	Low mood; masturbating to porn
	Childhood sexual abuse	Linda: Mummies don't cry	CSA and its impact in adulthood
		Elsie's care of her mother	The pain of accepting CSA
	Child sexual exploitation	Jade's struggle	Attempts to survive CSE
		Jaz: Keeping herself safe?	CSE denial
		Chloe's normal	Displaced anger disrupting intimacy and trust
	FGM	Furah: In pain	Type 3 infibulation; non-consummation
		Dr Tanous: Wrapped up	Displaced anger disrupting intimacy and trust
Reproductive years	Teenage pregnancy	Lucy and her twins	Teenage pregnancy
		Vicky's surprise	Unknown pregnancy
		Ava's need	Addressing risk
	Contraceptive provision	Bleeding Anna	No suitable method
		Tina and Levi: Double Dutch	Failed erection when using condoms
	Pregnancy	Sandra and Adam: Over- and under-prepared	Academic: practical and emotional challenges

(*Continued*)

(Continued)

Chapter	Section	Title of case study	Condition
Losses in reproductive years		Joanne: A ruined moment	Seventh pregnancy
		Heather's stem distraction	Cut off from intimacy
	Termination of pregnancy	Eve's hidden grief	Loss of sexual desire
	Infertility	Mike: A carriage of injustice	Erectile dysfunction
	Miscarriage	Serena's sadness	Loss of sexual desire
		Emily: When reassurance becomes painful	Painful sex
	Disruption of childbirth	Raj and Jen: Not seen but heard	Raj's fear of sex after childbirth
		Unreachable Rosie	Vaginismus
Unexpected outcomes	Near-death experiences and stillbirth	Jamie's terror	TOP and stillbirth
		Nuala's mourning	Loss of sexual desire
	Physical difference	Julie and Sam's protective love	Less than perfect baby: sex on hold
	Physical and mental challenges	Mo: Shouting to be heard	Relationship difficulties
		Lisa's love life	Sexuality confusion
	Acquired physical disability	Steph and Terry: Steph's secret	Terry's lack of awareness after his head injury; poor sexual experience for partner
		Marion's cover	Loss of desire: not felt sexy since her stroke
	Learning-disabled challenges	A good night out	A group formed by learning-disabled people to form romantic relationships
Mental health	Obsessive Compulsive Disorder	Waiting for Sabrina	OCD impacting sex
	Anxiety and depression	Leila: Blinded to the evidence	Marital break-up: anxiety, low state
		Zenab: What good is a weekend away?	Loss of desire, low mood, feelings of hopelessness

(Continued)

x   Case studies

(Continued)

Chapter	Section	Title of case study	Condition
Gender identity, sexuality and difference in sexual desire	Autistic traits	Clive's misconnection	Aversion to touch; Asperger's Syndrome
		Lovely Leonard	Anxiety with relationships
	Gender identity	Jackie and Ichika: Cross-purposes	Transgender female to male with lesbian partner; partner's loss of sexual connection
		Richard's responsibility	Gender identity issues
		Androgynous Amy	Gender confusion: no sexual feeling
		Finding Felicity	Non-binary; gender fluid
	Sexual desire and differences in sexual expression	Andres' rebellion	Sexuality confusion
		Marco's mania	Chem sex; sexual curiosity
		Tony/Irene's turmoil	Transvestism; gender Identity
	Differences in sexual desire and arousal	Caroline and Rashid: A mothering mismatch	Differences in sexual desire
		Tired Tim	Erectile dysfunction and loss of sexual desire
	Polyamory	Ray, Dave and Heidi: Three is not always a crowd	Polyamory
		Phillipe and Imka: Facing two ways and more	Polyamory and bisexual desire
	Fetish/paraphilia	Dimitri: Feet first	Fetish/paraphilia
		Peeping Tom	Upskirting
	Asexuality	Mia's minefield	Asexuality
Sexual health	The sexual health consultation	Poor Maggie	Full SH screen
		Tyrone's silence	SH screen; safer-sex advice
	STI screening	Frank's fall	Disbelief of negative results
		Aiden's cover-up	Nocturnal emissions
	HIV	Anxious Assim	HIV and health anxiety
		Stuck Simon	HIV and health anxiety with OCD
		Precious' time	HIV-positive result

(Continued)

(Continued)

Chapter	Section	Title of case study	Condition
	Unexpected disclosures of abuse	Olivia's oral history	Oral rape
		Pavel's business trip	Male sexual assault
		Submissive Sheila	Domestic violence
Women's health	Cervical smear test	Tara's testing time	Procedure anxiety
		Lucia's release from pain	Painful sex
	Colposcopy and hysteroscopy	Katie's change of direction	Avoiding colposcopy; intimate examination
		Yvette's distorted view	Fear of sex following colposcopy
Marriage and civil partnership	Expectations	Anita: Breaking a fantasy	Non-consummation
		Mark and Mandy: Hurt and hurting	Vaginismus post-marriage
		Grant and Seb: Tied in knots	Loss of desire
Hidden loss		Safina and Abdul: Seeking Safina	Non-consummation
		Gary and Esther: Go Gary go	Rapid ejaculation
		Lizzie and James: Living with Lizzie	Unhappy falling pregnant after failed IVF
		Peter and Leo: Catching up with Dad	Erectile failure
		Harriet: Burying her baby	Sudden infant death
Mid-life	Menopause	Not so silly Lilly	Peri-menopausal
		Louise and Greg's new connection	Painful sex
	Andropause	Directing Derek	Low mood
		Damien: Past, present and future	Erectile failure
	Surgery and medical conditions	Eileen rising	Mastectomy
		End of life for Joseph	Prostate cancer

(Continued)

xii *Case studies*

(*Continued*)

Chapter	Section	Title of case study	Condition
	Losses and gains	Alan's search	Post-heart attack loss of manhood
		Gloria's gain	Painful sex
		Widowed Wendy	Loss of sexual pleasure
Older age	Adapting to later life	Beryl's bravery	Gynae procedure
		Framed Freda	Vaginal repair
	New challenges in old age	Reggie lets himself out	Risky, unsafe sex
		Miss G and Edith: Touched by Miss G	Repeat antidepressant request
Supervision	Supervision cases	Lovely Leonard	Anxiety with relationships: all too lovely
		Precious' time	HIV-positive result; not knowing what to do
		Peeping Tom	Upskirting triggers concern
	Professional boundaries for therapy	Ariel's annoyance	Trans female: contagious irritation and blame

Preface

Welcome to this book and its contents!

Have you ever wondered why sex goes wrong or doesn't feel as good as everyone says it is? We have discovered that myriad life events and experiences can affect sexual development, intimacy and sexual function. After many discussions at the end of long working days, we have chosen to invest our time and energy to illustrate the value of exploring sex across the lifespan and to lay bare our professional experiences that have facilitated our learning. We hope that this will serve to educate and inspire anyone with an interest in intimacy, sex and relationships, both personally and professionally.

Between us we have a wealth of clinical experience in providing healthcare to adults and young people from all walks of life, from diverse ethnicities and communities and with differing sexual experiences and perspectives. Over the years of contact with people in health and illness, we have discovered that individuals and couples with concerns about intimacy and sexual function do not speak out about its importance unless they are invited to do so.

We have found that the empathic relationship with the patient in the routine of everyday practice, along with the ability to interpret body language, is fundamental to developing essential psychosexual skills to address blocks to sexual function and enjoyment. Throughout this book we will illustrate the effectiveness of our developed approach as we lay bare and demystify the subject of intimacy, sex and relationship challenges and how barriers can be removed. Thanks to the trust of the people who have shared their vulnerability, we have developed our skills through raw experiences in practice, learning that allowing ourselves not to have immediate answers can be a great asset. The real-life anonymised encounters in this book may not give an example of every situation, but we hope there is enough to illustrate that our applied principles in practice can achieve a positive outcome.

Although readers may find that their own story, either professionally or personally, has similarities to those described here, we have ensured that case and composite studies are disguised to prevent any individual from being identified. If anyone should experience a personal response to what is written in this book and wishes to pursue professional help or further professional development, please see 'Professional training and support' in Chapter 13. Equally, not all readers will consider intimacy, sexual function and relationships to be relevant for health and social care providers to address, but we hope minds will be changed by the insights gained through the content we provide.

We use the term 'health professional' (HP) for anyone working in a health or social care environment, inclusive of doctors and nurses in acute or primary care, allied health professionals and their assistants, clinical psychologists, counsellors, psychotherapists and social carers. The term 'patient' represents the individual who is seeking help, which can often be replaced by the term 'client', 'person' or 'individual', depending on the setting. The pronouns 'he', 'she' and 'they' are interchangeable.

We reference the early works and experiential training of those who have had a profound influence on our professional development and whose work will be of continuing value in the future, as well as using more recent respected references and current websites. You will find fewer references as you progress through the book as accounts of clinical experience take over, illustrating valuable principles which can be applied to practice.

Due to our personal and professional experiences over the years, we have gained rich perspectives on hard to discuss, intimate matters. We write with the intention of speaking to our readers on equal terms, with the consideration that at any time the health professional can become the one who is in need of help in this area. Special thanks are due to all those who have risked sharing their emotional, physical, sexual and relationship reality with us. We also have a deep appreciation for all the earlier pioneers in this field, for their boldness and humility, as they challenged professional practice to address this important aspect of healthcare. Due to this legacy, we hope that the contents of this book continue to challenge and inspire improved experiences and outcomes for patients, HPs, friends and families.

We are most grateful to Charley for her creativity in the diagram designs. We thank Jen for her expertise and constant availability for technical support and regular reviewing of the manuscript. Further thanks go to Matt, Doug, Bryony, Jon, Amber and Joel for their insightful perspectives and Katie for her enthusiasm on the final read-through. We have valued the expertise of our editors and publisher. Special appreciation also finally goes to our patient partners, families and friends for their continued encouragement despite our long writing journey.

We have shared tears of laughter and good company over the writing of this book. As authors, we combined our knowledge and skills in composing the content. This was a novel team enterprise. We are glad to have had the freedom to argue over phrasing and description, which has brought renewed empathy and respect among ourselves and for others. At times we have been struck by the depth of revelation in these pages that in writing has strengthened our learning and provided a clear vision of how the challenge for change within this book will benefit others.

We suggest that you dive into this book to widen your understanding of intimacy, sex and relationship challenges through the lifespan. By laying bare our successes and failures, readers will gain a deeper understanding of tried and tested ways of hearing and responding to intimate subjects with greater confidence.

Please join us on the journey of discovery.

Abbreviations and clarification of terms

Abbreviation	Terminology	Explanation
A&E	Accident and Emergency	Hospital department dealing with serious or life-threatening emergencies
AN/PN care	Antenatal/postnatal care	Care during pregnancy/care after the birth
ASD	Autistic Spectrum Disorder	DSM-5 categorises ASD as a neurodevelopmental disorder. There may be significant difficulties in social interaction and interpreting non-verbal communication, along with restricted and repetitive patterns of behaviour and interests. Three levels are suggested. Rather than 'disorder', the term 'neurodifferent' or 'neurodiverse' may be more helpful to individuals and families
BASHH		British Association for Sexual Health and HIV
	Cervical/intraepithelial lesion	A pre-cancerous lesion
	Cervical screening (cervical smear test)	A procedure to check the health of the cervix (neck of the womb)
	Cervix	The opening to the uterus (womb) from the vagina
Chem sex		Sexual enhancement through the use of chemical substances

(*Continued*)

(*Continued*)

Abbreviation	Terminology	Explanation
	Colposcopy	A procedure to look at the cervix and cervical os (entrance to the womb), often performed when cervical screening reveals abnormal cervical cells
	Commercial sex worker	Women, men and transgendered people who receive money or goods in exchange for sexual services and consciously define these activities as income generating even if they do not consider sex work as their occupation
CMHT	Community mental health team	CMHTs support people living in the community who have complex and/or serious mental health problems. Various mental health professionals work in CMHTs, including psychiatrists, psychologists, community psychiatric nurses, social workers and occupational therapists
	Consent to intimate examination	A patient must be given enough information and the offer of a chaperone to give their informed permission before any intimate examination is performed
	Contraception implant	A small flexible plastic rod placed under the skin in the upper arm by a doctor or nurse that releases the hormone progestogen into the bloodstream to prevent pregnancy (e.g. Nexplanon). Usually lasts for three years
	County lines	Drug-trafficking gangs who use non-traceable, temporary, 'pay as you go' phones to move drugs from one area to another

(*Continued*)

xviii *Abbreviations and clarification of terms*

(*Continued*)

Abbreviation	Terminology	Explanation
CS	Caesarean section	Also known as C-section. An operation to undertake the non-vaginal delivery of a baby
CSA	Childhood sexual abuse	There are two main types of childhood sexual abuse – contact and non-contact. Childhood sexual abuse can happen in person or online. Contact abuse is where an abuser makes physical sexual contact with a child after 'grooming'. Non-contact abuse may be the use of age-inappropriate sexual language, personal sexual reference, coercion into viewing pornographic images or being obliged to watch people engaging in sexual activity
CSE	Child sexual exploitation	A type of sexual abuse. When a child or young person is exploited they are given things like gifts, drugs, money, status and affection in exchange for performing sexual activities
	De-infibulation	A surgical procedure to reopen the vaginal entrance of women living with Type 3 FGM
DSM-5	*The Diagnostic and Statistical Manual of Mental Disorders*	Manual that is the product of more than ten years of effort by hundreds of international experts in all aspects of mental health

(*Continued*)

(Continued)

Abbreviation	Terminology	Explanation
ED	Erectile dysfunction	Getting and maintaining an erection adequate for penetration is a common problem. If the condition does not improve over three to six months, it is important to consult a GP for physical investigation. ED is more common after the age of forty but it can also be the result of thoughts, feelings and close relationships at any age. Sex therapy can be very helpful
	Epidural	Spinal block – an anaesthetic injection into the epidural space
	Fetish/paraphilia	Intense sexual arousal relating to atypical objects, situations, fantasies, behaviours, individuals or body parts
FGM	Female genital mutilation	All procedures involving the partial or total removal of the external female genitalia or any other injury to female genital organs for non-medical reasons (infibulation). Four types are described
FSH screen	Full sexual health screen	Screen carried out in a Genito-Urinary Medicine (GUM) clinic, which may include taking swabs, blood and urine for testing
FSRH		Faculty of Reproductive and Sexual Healthcare, England (FSRH)
	Gender fluid	A person whose gender identity is not personally felt to be either male or female. The experienced gender identity may fluctuate over time

(Continued)

Abbreviations and clarification of terms

(Continued)

Abbreviation	Terminology	Explanation
	Gender incongruence	When the emotional and psychological identity as male or female is opposite or different from the biological sex, which therefore feels alien or unacceptable to the individual
GP	General practitioner (also known as primary care physician)	Registered with the General Medical Council (England)
HIV	Human Immunodeficiency Virus	A virus that is transmitted through contact with infected semen or vaginal fluids during unprotected vaginal, anal or oral sex
HP	Health professional	As defined in the UK, a health professional is a person associated with either a specialty or a discipline and who is qualified and allowed by regulatory bodies to provide a healthcare service to a patient
HV	Health visitor	A qualified registered nurse or midwife who has completed a course in specialist community public health nursing or health visiting approved by the Community Practitioners and Health Visitors Association (CPHVA)
	Hymen	A membrane which partially crosses the opening of the vagina
	Hysteroscopy	Examination of the inside of the uterus (womb) by the insertion of a slim tube with a tiny light and camera to look for the causes of symptoms

(Continued)

Abbreviations and clarification of terms xxi

(*Continued*)

Abbreviation	Terminology	Explanation
	Infibulation	The practice of excising the clitoris and labia of a girl or woman and stitching together the edges of the vulva to prevent sexual intercourse. Traditional in some cultures but highly controversial and now against the law in the UK
	Intimate physical examination	An examination of breasts, genitalia (internal or external) and rectal area (internal or external)
IVF	In-vitro fertilisation	An egg is removed from the woman's ovaries and fertilised with a sperm in the laboratory. The embryo (fertilised egg) is returned to the woman's uterus (womb) to grow and develop
	Mastectomy	A surgical operation to remove a breast
	Menopause	Officially marks the end of female reproduction: i.e. the natural cessation of monthly bleeds (periods)
	Miscarriage of pregnancy	Loss of a pregnancy usually before twenty weeks' gestation
'MUS'	Medically unexplained symptoms	This is a wide term for a number of medically investigated persistent physical symptoms of over six months' duration with no known medical cause; however, it often refers to the most severe type but much fewer in number, known as Somatic Symptom Disorder (DSM-5), which can disrupt everyday life and mental wellbeing over many years

(*Continued*)

(Continued)

Abbreviation	Terminology	Explanation
	Non-binary	A broad spectrum of gender identities that are not exclusively masculine or feminine
NSPCC	National Society for the Prevention of Cruelty to Children	The UK's leading children's charity, preventing abuse and helping those affected to recover
OC	Oral contraception	Includes combined oral contraception (COC), progestogen only pill (POP) and emergency contraception pill (ECP)
OCD	Obsessive Compulsive Disorder	Usually a particular pattern of repeated negative thoughts and behaviour
O&G	Obstetrics and gynaecology	Field of medicine that deals with pregnancy, childbirth and women's health
	Parentcraft classes	Knowledge of antenatal, delivery and postnatal care delivered within health or social care settings by NHS, third sector or private providers
	Patient	'The one who is suffering' and seeking help, interchangeable with 'client' or 'service user'; reference to 'he' or 'she' ('his/hers') is interchangeable with 'they' ('their')
	PDE-5i	A group of medicines that can be used to treat ED
	Performance anxiety	Caused by negative thoughts about the ability to perform well during sexual activity
	Peri-menopausal	The start of menopausal symptoms caused by the drop in oestrogen through to the end of ovulation cycles
	Polyamory	Engaging in multiple sexual relationships with the consent of all involved

(Continued)

Abbreviations and clarification of terms xxiii

(Continued)

Abbreviation	Terminology	Explanation
	Pre- and post-menopausal	The stage before the menstrual cycle becomes irregular and the stage after all menstruation has ceased, respectively
PrEP	Pre-exposure prophylaxis	The taking of medication by an HIV-negative person to prevent HIV transmission prior to potential exposure
	Psychosexual issues	Examples include vaginismus (painful vaginal penetration), anorgasmia, loss of sexual desire, premature ejaculation, delayed ejaculation, erectile failure and sex addiction
	Psychosexual therapist/counsellor	In the UK training to become a psychosexual therapist is validated by the College of Sexual and Relationship Therapists (COSRT), generally for already trained relationship counsellors but may also be undertaken by experienced qualified nurses, doctors and other trained counsellors; alternatively, registered healthcare professionals may have additional training from the Institute of Psychosexual Medicine (IPM) or previous experiential training under the quality standards of the former Association of Psychosexual Nursing, alongside extensive clinical experience
PST	Psychosexual therapy	The therapist engages with the individual through an agreed therapy contract to address personal goals concerning sexual function, sexual distress, sexuality and sometimes gender identity issues

(Continued)

xxiv *Abbreviations and clarification of terms*

(*Continued*)

Abbreviation	Terminology	Explanation
RE/PE	Rapid/premature ejaculation	Ejaculating too early during sexual intercourse
R&R model	Reflect and Respond model	Our approach to learning from practice: reflecting honestly on what has happened and choosing to take the learning forward into subsequent consultations
	Sexting	The sharing of sexually explicit personal photographs or videos or sexually explicit messaging over the internet often via a mobile electronic device
	Sexual fantasy	An erotic yearning or grouping of mental images that bring about sexual arousal
	Sexual health history taking	Recording intimate details of a patient's sexual history to determine the optimum course of action in terms of examination, laboratory investigation and treatment
SG	Safeguarding procedures (local)	Multi-disciplinary organisational protocols for the protection of children and vulnerable adults
SH clinic	Sexual health clinic	Provides testing, treatment and advice about sexually transmitted infections. May also offer contraceptive care
SHA	Sexual health advisor	Professional (usually a qualified nurse, health visitor, social worker or counsellor) who provides information, advice and counselling in a sexual health clinic to patients who have been diagnosed with a sexually transmitted infection. The SHA plays a key role in helping the patient understand the transmission, treatment and management of their condition

(*Continued*)

Abbreviations and clarification of terms xxv

(*Continued*)

Abbreviation	Terminology	Explanation
SIDS	Sudden Infant Death Syndrome	The sudden, unexpected and unexplained death of an apparently healthy baby; previously could be referred to as 'cot death'
	Social services	A range of public services provided by the government to support vulnerable families, children and adults
	Stem cells	Cells taken from an embryo, umbilical cord or an adult that are used for treating blood disorders such as leukaemia and the repair of other organs
STI	Sexually transmitted infection	Examples of STIs are chlamydia, gonorrhoea, genital warts, genital herpes, syphilis and HIV
STI screening	Sexually transmitted infection screening	Routine screening for sexually transmitted infections
TOP	Termination of pregnancy	Ending a pregnancy by medication and/or mechanical means
	Transgender	When a person's sense of personal gender identity does not correspond with their birth/biological sex
	Transvestism	The practice of dressing and acting in a style or manner traditionally associated with the opposite sex, sometimes but not always with high sexual arousal
	Umbilical cord prolapse	The umbilical cord comes out of the uterus (womb) with or before the presenting part of the baby which can compromise blood flow to the baby

(*Continued*)

(Continued)

Abbreviation	Terminology	Explanation
uPPS	Unresolved persistent physical symptoms	This term, developed through a research journey into MUS, identifies the largest group seeking help for persistent physical symptoms not getting better over time nor with routine medical care including persistent sexual dysfunctions which may be helped by talking therapy interventions
	Vaginismus	When the band of muscle approximately 2.5cm (1 inch) into the vagina suddenly tightens up just as something is inserted into it. Painful and distressing, but can be treated
	Wellbeing service	An Improving Access to Psychological Therapy (IAPT) UK government initiative to provide easily accessible, evidence-based treatments for those experiencing common mental health problems, such as anxiety, depression, OCD, etc.
	Youth gang culture	Mostly street-based groups of young people for whom crime and violence is an essential part of the group's identity

Introduction

How did we get here?

> I felt shocked and sad after my shift that day and I wanted to understand why and what had affected me that way. The couple were so intimate and loving but had never had sexual intercourse in their ten-year relationship … and they had just had a baby!
>
> (See 'Unreachable Rosie', Chapter 3)

The statement above is an example of how the desire to learn more about the skills needed to talk to patients about such intimate matters can be triggered. Over years of training and working with sexual anxieties in various acute and community healthcare settings, we noticed a common theme: people do not bring up the subject of sex and intimacy unless they are given a clear signal to do so. Furthermore, health professionals often lack confidence in addressing the many aspects of sexuality, gender and sexual function of those in their care. This subject is little mentioned in health and social care training curricula, nor in practice, despite many recognising the sexual concerns of individuals within their specialisms (Rani, 2009; Moore, 2009; Heath and White, 2002).

For those people who frequently attend services seeking help with persistent medically unresolved sexual dysfunction, repeated medical tests can potentially feed their anxiety and exacerbate physical and mental distress. Furthermore, when sexual development or sexual function becomes difficult or impossible at any point in the lifespan, it can be the cause of personal confusion and upset. How can we acknowledge and develop insights and understanding to support individuals or couples or ourselves to work through these difficulties? An accessible approach to start to answer this challenging question is shared in the following chapters through the personal and professional reflections, confusions, delights and dilemmas across our lifetimes of healthcare practice.

The anonymised and composite cases that we share illustrate the need for a sensitive approach. In therapy we pause to think about what is happening in the moment and by doing this a focused response can be developed with each person. Our Reflect and Respond model (R&R), which is demonstrated later, shows this reflective process in action. This model sits well within a co-equal therapeutic relationship between the health professional (HP) and the patient, which is essential when addressing sexual matters and contrasts with the expectation of all parties that someone else with the expertise will 'fix the problem'.

The previously undisputed aim of all HPs has been to treat, care and cure, or at least 'to make it better' and ultimately 'do no harm'. This surely also applies to individuals and couples who want to 'make it better' at home but end up not talking about what matters for fear of hurting each other. In the healthcare environment, along with the added time pressures of healthcare delivery, the R&R approach may be beneficial as a way of achieving better outcomes.

It is important when engaging with this subject area to resist the temptation to resort to professional instruction or good ideas, which do not necessarily help the individual to discover the heart of the matter for themselves. Sitting back, putting a pen down, pushing a keyboard away and listening carefully to the evidence helps to avoid slipping into professional expertise. However, even for a moment, this can represent a challenge for a well-trained HP, as it may require moving into unfamiliar territory.

Training and applied principles

We have developed our psychosexual awareness and skills using the psychoanalytic perspectives of Michael and Enid Balint, applied to general practice and social work from the early 1950s (Balint and Balint, 1961). Since the early 1970s Balint-style seminars have also been used to facilitate training for nurses and other HPs in addressing sexual difficulties in practice, under the guidance of the former Association of Psychosexual Nursing, inaugurated in 1998 (Wells, 2000; Irwin, 2011). The study of the practitioner–patient relationship within a clinical encounter in the routine of everyday practice lies at the heart of the experiential psychosexual skills training seminars. This guiding principle was in common with the training provided by the Institute of Psychosexual Medicine (IPM). Concerning intimate matters, the work of the IPM enhances HP–patient encounters and is underpinned by the reflections and principles of psychoanalysts Malan and Main, the latter also a leading psychiatrist involved with the mental health community, Cassel Hospital, London,

UK. Both, amongst others, outlined the potential of brief psychotherapy and the value of sharing these broad principles with medical, nursing and social work colleagues (Balint, 1964; Malan, 1976; Main, 1989). This method of ongoing reflection, supervision and training enables a tailored response to the individual to good and timely effect as he or she presents with psychosexual anxieties within the clinical environment (Penman, 2009; Burridge, 2017).

In general, those in caring professions seek to solve an issue, put it right or remove the cause of suffering. In this way we can readily step into the expert role, instruct, give advice which has worked with others, and then feel satisfied with our intervention. Equally, with relief, we may quickly refer on to another specialist if one is available. And the patient? What do they feel? (See Figure 0.1.)

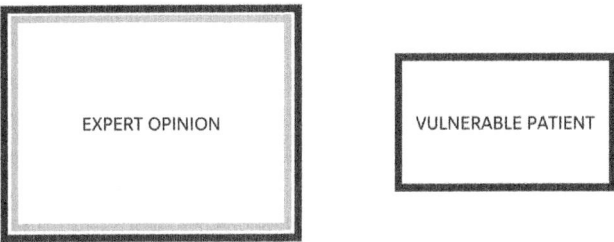

Figure 0.1 The expert and the patient. Source: Penman, 1998

The person who takes the 'expert' position on the subject of sexual dysfunction and intimacy may leave the patient without a voice, vulnerable and frustrated. The 'expert' in this instance is usually thanked but there is no essential personal change. If we do not consider that we have a professional competence to address intimate issues, we may naturally adopt the comforting and reassuring role, encouraging that all will be well soon enough (see Figure 0.2).

The instinct to enfold with comfort and reassurance ensures the individual has little chance to speak out. The truth of personal experience may be suffocated; there may be a feeling of gratitude for the comfort and care, but the opportunity to address such a sensitive subject can so easily be lost (Penman, 1998).

As the HP attempts to make it safer for the person to share uncertain and difficult feelings they may fear that this will open up issues beyond their particular clinical expertise; a fear of lengthening and complicating any routine intervention in already overstretched services thereby

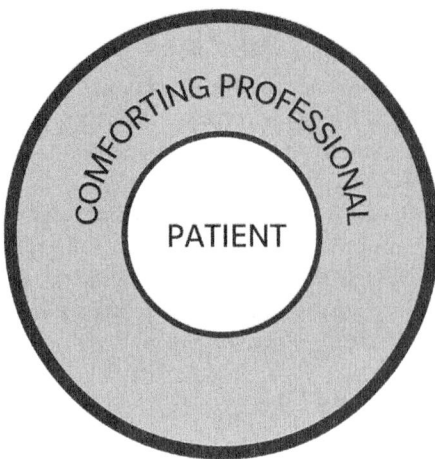

Figure 0.2 The comforter. Source: Penman, 1998

becomes a barrier to change. Conversely, we and others working in the way we outline in this book, rather than providing ready-made solutions, have found through experience that facilitating the sharing of sensitive information can both enhance and shorten the intervention with an improved outcome (Penman, Cook and Randhawa, 2020, Penman, 2019; Wells, 2000; Skrine, 1997).

As you will see in our Reflect and Respond model, demonstrated in later chapters, we offer a view into an effective therapeutic HP–patient relationship for addressing very intimate matters (outlined in more detail in Figures 0.3 and 0.4). This adjusted relationship moves away from the role of expert HP with all the answers and from the role of comforter. After investigations have not revealed any currently known medical condition, in these difficult circumstances, we have found that more may be achieved with the patient by a joint 'unknowing' and exploration of what the body may be doing and why. In parallel, the door must always remain open to further medical investigation, as required.

The Reflect and Respond model

The Reflect and Respond model (R&R) emerges from professional reflective practice supporting a focus on the task in hand. Reflective practice has been used for many years in health and social care settings in order to develop self-awareness and to improve practice process and outcomes over time (Bond and Holland, 1998). This type of evidence from reflective practice supports the findings of evidence-based practice in the discovery of what matters to the individual for effective care (Schwandt, 2002; Tonelli, 2001).

This simple R&R tool enables us to reflect in and on practice (Schön, 1983), in the moment and later, and to personalise our responses to the individual as we engage in the unpredictability of human relationships. This enables the possibility to capture rich practice-based findings using reflexivity to gather learning from the anonymised and subjectively experienced material whilst ensuring crucial confidentiality (Etherington, 2004). Our first example of the R&R model can be found in the case of Celine in Chapter 1.

The R&R process starts with listening and absorbing the practical and emotional information that the individual conveys when seeking help. In complex human circumstances, a standard input does not necessarily result in an expected outcome. As we think about how best to use our professional selves, we try to let go of our preconceived notions of what works, from past experience.

The therapeutic opportunity develops over moments in time. Now, the individual seeking help and the HP are co-equal. This adjusted 'point of view' allows an active engagement with the previously unexplored body responses. As the individual's insights and personal resources for change are facilitated by the HP, it is possible to trust the concept of 'not knowing' the answer. This is enabled within the protected and non-judgemental space, resulting in increasing self-understanding and the option of personal choice as to what may help moving forward. The connections between body, mind and emotion become clearer to both parties during and between consultations through this jointly developed trust. In addition, the potential for improved intimacy is enhanced.

The co-production of a creative, safe therapeutic space allows for uncertainty, open-minded exploration and improved experience.

Once the HP's skills are developed through experience and supervised practice, we have found substantial benefits and witnessed improved therapeutic outcomes for sufferers. In view of this, our aim is to take time to build confidence by encouraging other HPs to understand the importance and value of listening to a patient's sexual and relationship concerns relevant to their health and wellbeing.

We reflect on how the individual perceives the problem or concern and on what they hope to get from the consultation on that day. From this starting point, we begin to cooperate on their terms rather than our own and to respond to the individual in a way that is specific to their particular need. As we do this, we can return to the unique evidence communicated either directly or indirectly from the sufferer's personal account. Through this humane professional response, we grow in sensitivity and respect as we reflect together on the consequences of their context. In using this approach, attending to the layers of communication, the discovery of what matters and the joint interpretation all build a broader picture of the context of the difficulty. With experience and skill, the process can begin within the time available to address the medically unresolved concerns – in this case, concerning intimate matters.

The R&R model allows for unexpected insights to be shared in the therapeutic space. (See Figure 0.3). Often, the reality of body, mind and emotional expression within a safe space develops a conscious awareness of the numerous influences on physical health and sexual function. In this way, the individual is empowered to decide in which direction they need to go. Therefore, not only does the 'Reflect' component allow space for the individual to grow in personal insight but the 'Respond' attitude enables respectful cooperation and enhanced ownership and insight over the best way forward. Our own physical and emotional responses may also lead to professional and personal revelation and learning.

The R&R model can be used further to record the process of individual learning as continuing professional development. The following form (Table 0.1) has been developed for this purpose. It may be used only with the accompanying acknowledgement.

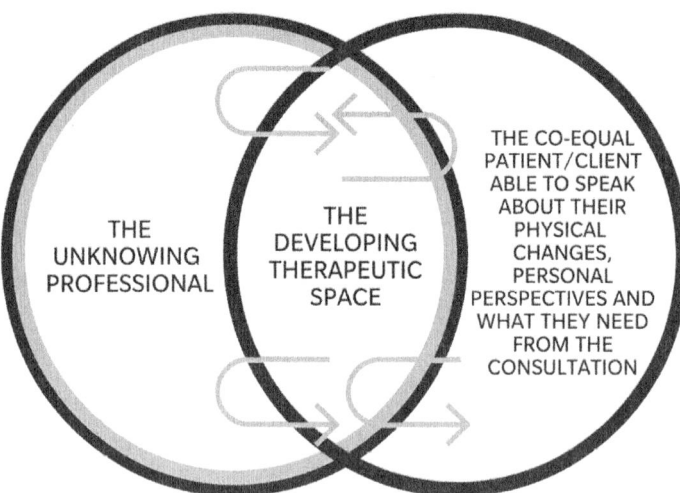

Figure 0.3 The therapeutic space developed through the practitioner–patient relationship. Source: Penman, 1998

Table 0.1 Reflect and Respond model process template: recording learning and practice development

Date:	Role:	Initials:
REFLECT	What is the issue?	
	How did the encounter go: beginning, middle and end?	
	What part did I play: verbally, practically, emotionally?	
	What was the outcome?	
	How did this reflection help me to understand the patient and myself better?	
RESPOND	What could I do differently next time?	
	How will I share my findings with colleagues?	

Source: Benns, Burridge and Penman, 2021

When used regularly for debriefing in protected time, the R&R process builds practice-based knowledge which is not always recognised by individuals or shared in teams. It allows for success and failure to be examined, reduces shame, builds confidence, develops humility and strengthens cooperation when addressing complex issues in practice.

As you read on, we will illustrate how the model is used to expose and examine interactions and improve outcomes in the real-world encounters of our experience. In the next section you will see that we start to focus on demystifying the subject of intimacy, sex and relationship challenges by providing a broad explanation of the terms used in the book.

Finding the heart of the matter

In our experience the presenting sexual problem for each person, following the exclusion of any organic cause, is often the unique expression of hidden disruption and buried distress. We have found that psychosexual difficulties, which are a result of body/mind and emotional influences, may be underpinned by some of the experiences illustrated in Figure 0.4.

As this figure illustrates, the underlying factors are endless. In our experience, people can also suffer not only with persistent sexual symptoms (longer than six months' duration) but also other forms of persistent 'medically unexplained' ill health or physical dysfunction. 'Medically unexplained symptoms' (MUS) is now considered a largely unhelpful term (Sharpe, 2013). Many healthy physical responses automatically come into play to protect the individual from further harm and to assist healing, but if a threat is still perceived, the body's systems may still be on high alert. This can cause very real physical problems, including sexual, if the automatic self-protecting sexual responses remain, leading to much

8 Introduction

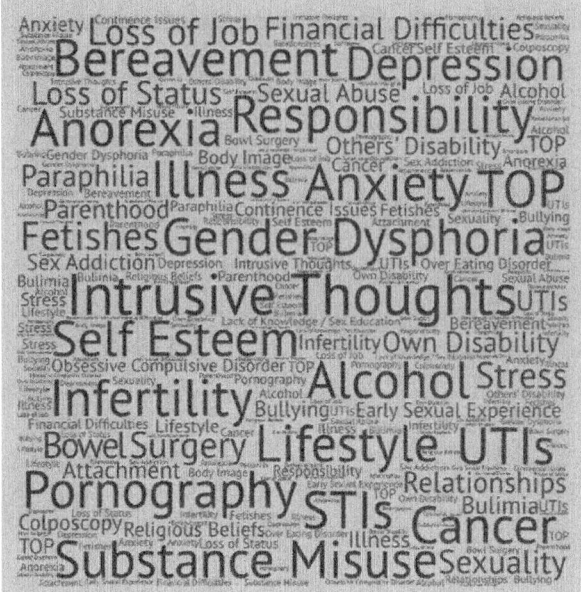

Figure 0.4 Finding the heart of the matter: underpinning factors which may be found when talking to people with sexual dysfunction or sexual dissatisfaction

frustration over things not improving for everyone involved. Often, in such instances, despite thorough investigation, no currently known disease-based cause can be found (Nimnuan, Hotopf and Wessely, 2001). This can be the case and is commonly observed when there is no improvement with usual primary care or specialist medical care interventions, with the temptation to ascribe the physical dysfunction as 'all in the head'. We have discovered this not to be true.

Much of the important inside connections between body, mind and emotion can now be explained by the work of psycho-neuro-biological researchers (e.g. Hellhammer and Hellhammer, 2008; Watkins, 1997) as understandable physiological events in response to a particular personal context. In a study of psychosexual counselling process, persistent sexual symptoms were also found to be aligned with some of the predisposing factors for 'MUS' that are highlighted in the literature (Penman, 2015). The study of the therapy process showed a number of common themes across the therapy process in reducing or resolving the negative impact of medically unresolved persistent physical symptoms (uPPS) – a term which emerged through and following the evaluation research process (see Figure 0.5; Penman, 2015, 2018).

An exploration of precipitating factors in the development of an identified sexual problem can provide an insight into why the problem started. Emotions that are triggered by life events can often be expressed as sexual dysfunction (see Peter and Leo's case study in Chapter 10). At this point, there appears to be no conscious awareness of any link between previous life events and the current difficulty. A mutually developed understanding of the history and continuing concerns provides a personalised way forward. At times when the links between body, mind and emotion become conscious, the speed of physical recovery can be breathtaking (see Emily's case study in Chapter 3).

We suggest that the solutions to personal sexual 'dysfunctions' or 'disorders' may not lie solely in textbooks. Rather, the resolution of many persistent sexual difficulties comes from the exploration and discoveries

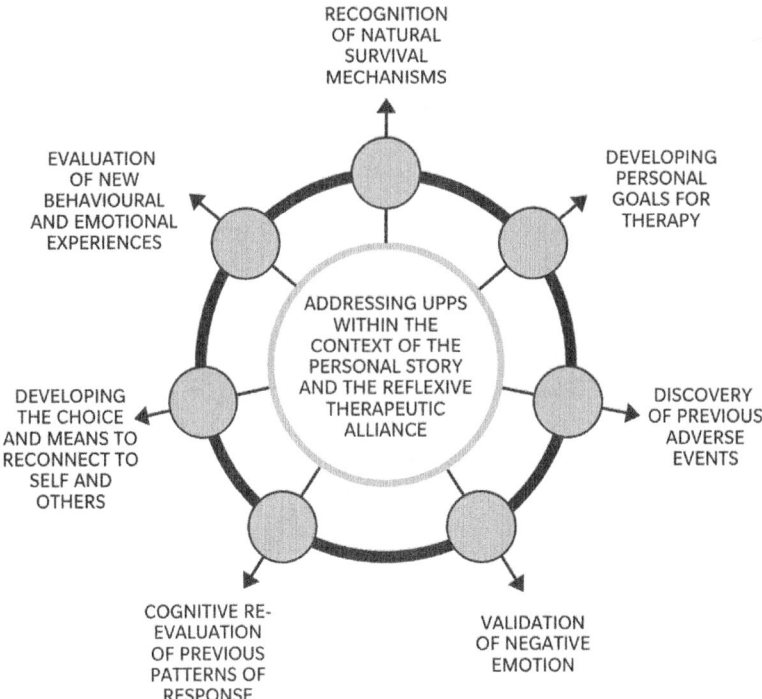

Figure 0.5 Therapy process: themes discovered during an intervention for reducing persistent sexual symptoms. Source: Penman, 2015

made between the HP and the context of the individual: their environment and relationships, past and present experiences, future hopes and fears. This perspective on sex and intimacy concerns has also been acknowledged by other psychosexual therapists writing in an accessible way on female sexual difficulties relevant to male and female and gender non-binary readers (Nagoski, 2015; Gurney, 2020).

What's it all about?

Frequently, people simply want to know 'Am I normal'? or to discover what is wrong with them (see Celine's case study in Chapter 1). In our clinical practice, we remain open, within the confines of the law, to each individual's interpretation, gender, sexual preferences and motivation as to what is 'normal' for them. It is listening to the context of the individual's real-world experience and their sexual preferences that allows for honesty and respect within the HP–patient relationship from the beginning. In this section we begin to explore motivation for sex, sexual attraction, asexuality, sexual dysfunction and sex and gender identity.

People differ in their experience of sexual practice and intimacy and some may prefer one without the other. There is no one definition that covers all sexual expression. For example, in Western culture, Valins (1992: p. 127) described how sexuality had become directed towards the masculine goal of intercourse and orgasm. Valins continued to suggest that the myth conveyed by films and pornography that women want 'hard, aggressive and fast sexual intercourse' could lead to misunderstandings between sexual partners. However, today there is a recognition in society that it is acceptable for women to be more sexually assertive and to know what they want. Nevertheless, in any kind of sexual relationship there can be confusion and unrealistic expectations.

Valins argued that intercourse is not just a sexual event, but can be expanded to embrace one's body, mind, heart and spirit. Hall, writing on treating sex addiction and the need to strengthen intimacy, concludes that intimacy can be difficult to define but for 'most couples this is the aspect of their relationship that can bring most fulfilment' (Hall, 2013: p.151). Hall suggests that intimacy is built on communication and relates broadly to six categories: emotional, physical, intellectual, spiritual, lifestyle and recreation.

We will now uncover some of the sexual terms used within this book, although it is not our intention to give detailed definitions of sexual practices. Rather, we begin by thinking about sexual attraction and why people may be motivated to have sex.

Sexual attraction and motivation

The basic biological drive for sexual activity is found in the majority of human populations. Some people have lifelong attraction to the opposite or same sex; however, others may change during the lifespan due to innumerable health, social, environmental, cultural, ethical and/or spiritual factors. There are many other terms, such as 'pansexual', meaning that biological sex is not the first consideration for experiencing an attraction. In sexual health settings it is important to know about sexual orientation and sexual partners because this can impact on the health advice required.

Living in same-sex organisations such as schools, religious establishments or prisons can lead to sexual activity with those in close proximity for that period in time, but neuro-plasticity (human adaptability) may enable subsequent reversion to a previous sexual attraction and activity. Some people may continue with a bisexual attraction. There are likely to be many descriptions of sexual attraction preferences, but these are beyond the scope of this book.

Figure 0.6 illustrates some of the social, emotional, financial, health and other motivations for sex that we have encountered.

Asexuality

A small minority of people are not interested in the physical aspect of sexual activity, although they may seek a romantic relationship. However, others do not want either. The Asexual Visibility & Education Network (AVEN) defines asexuality as: 'not having sexual feelings towards others: not experiencing sexual desire or attraction. In general, an asexual person does not feel or otherwise experience any sexual attraction' (Merriam-Webster, n.d.). This absence of sexual desire may be inborn, but we have found that it is sometimes acquired through negative experiences.

In the next section we define some of the terms that you will encounter later in this book, including sexual dysfunctions and the biological, genetic and social components of sex and gender identity.

Defining a sexual dysfunction

It has been suggested that the first three elements in the following list (not necessarily in order) are required for a 'successful' sexual response, so when sex goes wrong the problem may be categorised under these general terms:

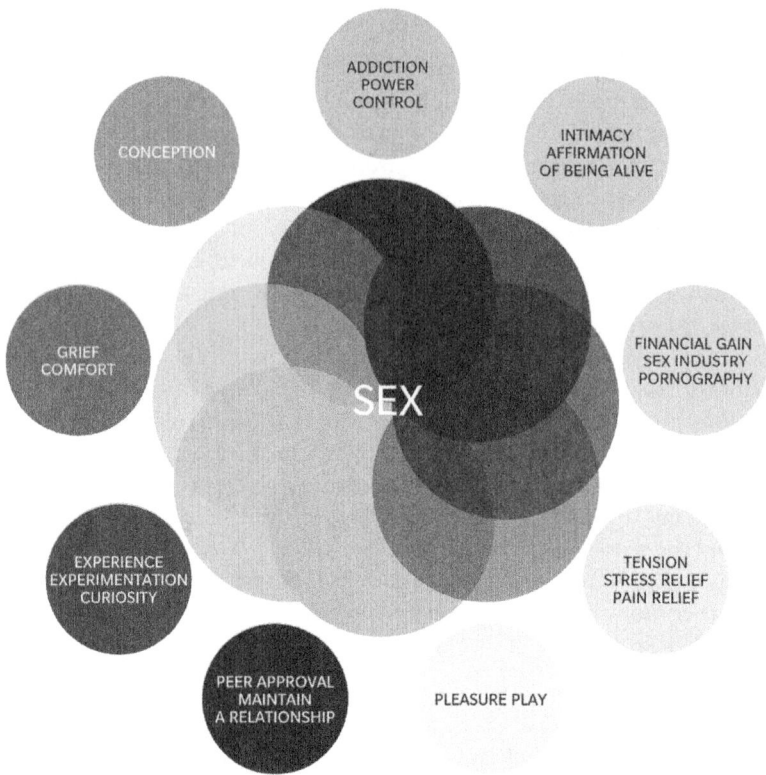

Figure 0.6 Examples of physical and emotional motivations for sex and intimacy

- Desire: motivation for sexual activity
- Arousal: mental and physical changes in response to sexual activity
- Orgasm: pleasurable physical and mental response to sexual stimulation
- Pain: thoughts of sexual activity, actual sexual stimulation or penetration causing physical pain

Psychosexual therapy professionals such as Nagoski (2015) and Gurney (2020) emphasise that for many women the desire for sex often emerges only once sexual arousal has begun. Furthermore, not all women require orgasm on each occasion to feel the benefit of physical intimacy. These realities need to be appreciated when seeking to understand a sexual problem, anxiety or concern.

The diagnosis of sexual dysfunction is classified under a specific mental health category within the *Diagnostic Statistical Manual of Mental Disorders* (DSM-5) (American Psychiatric Association, 2013). Concerns of disrupted desire, arousal, orgasm and genital pain become quantified as technical and mental disorders in order to receive health insurance funding for treatment, but also to encourage international research into specific conditions diagnosed using the manual's guidance. Conditions are separated by further description (see the list below).

DSM-5 diagnostic categories for sexual dysfunction

- Female Genito-Pelvic Pain/Penetration Disorder, inclusive of vaginismus and dyspareunia (males have no equivalent in DSM-5 for genital pain as insufficient research has been conducted in this area to create a diagnostic category)
- Delayed Ejaculation
- Premature Ejaculation
- Female Sexual Interest/Arousal Disorder
- Male Hypoactive Sexual Desire Disorder
- Female Orgasmic Disorder
- Erectile Disorder
- Substance/Medication Induced Sexual Dysfunction
- Other Specified Sexual Disorder
- Unspecified Sexual Disorder

Following discussion with the individual, these conditions are qualified by the attending HP as:

- Lifelong/acquired
- Generalised/situational
- Distress: mild/moderate/severe

Such examples of sexual dysfunction classification, as defined by DSM-5, show how the inevitable complexity and nuance of human sexual relationships and physical sexual expression are largely set aside during diagnosis. These defined conditions have caused concern for many because they are found within the mental health section. Linked to this is the importance of understanding whether the terms 'Gender Dysphoria' and 'Gender Identity Disorder' are acceptable to either HPs or their patients. The International Classification of Diseases (ICD) is used more commonly than the DSM worldwide, but there have been efforts to harmonise the two systems. To this end, a group of specialists were assembled to update ICD 10 to ICD 11 (WHO, n.d.). As with all updating processes regarding classification, attempts were made to understand and develop further clarity around individuals' gender identity challenges (WHO Regional Office for Europe, n.d.). Consequently, 'Gender Incongruence' is now the generally accepted term for what was previously known as 'Gender Dysphoria' or 'Gender Identity Disorder', and the condition has been moved out of the mental disorders section and placed within the sexual health section, thereby reducing the medicalisation of lived experience. It is also recognised that sexual dysfunctions and sexual pain disorders may be linked to other causes, such as medical conditions and their treatments, psychological factors, medications, relationship issues and cultural factors. We have found this confirmed in practice (see Figure 0.4).

The cases in the following chapters have not been strictly defined by the diagnostic classifications of either DSM-5 or ICD 11. However, the majority of these patients had experienced more than a year of substantial distress due to sexual dysfunction or gender identity difficulties, and neither time nor previous general or specialist medical intervention had improved matters for them.

Sex and gender identity

In the past, 'sex' and 'gender' were often used interchangeably, so these terms require clarification. Biological sex is usually determined by the appearance of the external genitalia and genetic testing for sex chromosomes if the physical signs at birth are uncertain. For the majority of any given population, the biological sex aligns with their gender identity as male or female (known by some as 'cisgender'). The development of gender identity is influenced by society's expectations. However, a child who does not or cannot meet the expectations of their gender role within their social environment is often ostracised, blamed or bullied for their difference. This creates a sense of not belonging to any group – male or female – leading to low self-esteem, social insecurity and subsequent low mood and anxiety. As part of human nature, we all seek a secure identity and a sense of belonging. In practice we are also seeing an increase in individuals with Autistic Spectrum Disorder traits with gender identity uncertainty, adding further complexity to their distress. In many cases, the motivation for changing the body to fit an internal gender identity is the hope to become more connected to themselves and others and to find their place in the world. We conclude that the motivation for physical gender change is rarely linked to sexual preference or desire.

Individuals who identify as non-binary – not wanting to be labelled with the expectations of a male or female gender identity – are not necessarily welcomed into transgender communities. People who identify as trans generally want to identify as male or female. Under UK law, all existing previous reference to birth sex is prohibited following gender change once personal documents have been formalised (although some individuals do not want to deny all of their past gender history). This can precipitate personal, emotional and healthcare screening dilemmas if the birth/biological sex is not known. Furthermore, due to the complexities, waiting times and high expectations of complete physical transition, for personal reasons the individual can be left frustrated and sometimes disappointed with the final result. This may lead to further body dysmorphia, mental health issues and, for a few, even suicidal feelings.

A small number of people may be born with biological evidence of both male and female reproductive organs, known as 'intersex'. Because the genitals of the baby are atypical, the birth sex is unclear. The sex of the baby is generally determined by a joint medical and parental decision, but over time this may be in opposition to the individual's personal developing gender identity. In this conflict, due to a sex chromosome abnormality, future surgery may be required for the individual to enjoy an alignment with their experienced gender identity.

There are circumstances in which an individual presents physically as male or female, but their sex chromosomes indicate the opposite due to abnormalities. This means the individual, through no fault of their own, may fail to develop in line with their sex chromosome indicators – XX for females and XY for males. An example of this conundrum is the debate in elite sport regarding the right of some athletes to compete in women's events. Female athletes have been banned due to abnormalities in their sex chromosomes causing higher than usual testosterone levels. This challenging situation has resulted in a heated debate over what constitutes 'cheating' and 'unfair advantage'. A glimpse into such complexities should lead us to further research and greater compassion for those who do not meet the expectations of society's sex and gender norms.

From an early age a minority of people who experience discontent with their gender role may seek pleasure and peace through cross-dressing in the opposite sex gender role in private. We have found that cross-dressing in private – which is not necessarily linked to sexual arousal – can provide sufficient relief for some individuals to maintain their expected gender role in public and in close relationships.

Gender incongruence

An increasing and unremitting hatred of biological sexual development and feelings of gender identity incongruence with the expected norms may lead to severe mental health issues. Studies have shown that gender incongruent people are twice as likely to have suicidal thoughts than lesbian, gay or bisexual people (Haas et al., 2011; McNeill, Ellis and Eccles, 2017; Centre for Suicide Prevention, n.d.). A 30-year Swedish clinical study that examined attempted or actual suicide rates 10–15 years after gender transition reported a rate that was 19 per cent higher than that in a similar demographic control group. The levels of cardiovascular disease and the development of neoplasms (a growth of cells that may be non-malignant, pre-cancerous or cancerous) following the use of sex hormones were also found to be raised (Batty, 2004). Of course, all such research findings demand close reading, and not enough is yet known regarding longer-term outcomes (Yüksel et al., 2017). For instance, the Swedish study requests more research into individuals' experience of physical gender transition at least ten years' post-transition, inclusive of emotional, mental and physical health. Further research in this field is vital to understand more about pre- and post-transition experiences so that equal access to healthcare is made available.

A person with a male biological sex who has an internal female gender identity is often known as 'trans female' or 'trans woman' (MtoF); and for a person of female biological sex with an internal male gender identity, the term 'trans male' or 'trans man' (FtoM) may be similarly acceptable. Due to increasing media coverage of changing gender to the binary opposite, many hundreds of people have recently come forward to request help in this area for the relief of distress and sometimes to demand life-changing treatments: adolescent blocking hormones, opposite sex hormones, or surgery to alter genitals, breasts and other body parts. Medical monitoring continues after transition, and must take any potential physical and mental health risks into account (Gender Identity Clinic, n.d.).

In adolescent gender reassignment services, many patients eventually decide not to transition, and some clinicians have argued that the hormonal blockers that delay puberty can be safely reversed. However, we do not yet have access to enough long-term research on the physical and emotional impact of puberty-blocking medications to warrant complete confidence in this area. Young people can find advice and guidance via the NHS's Gender Identity Development Service website (see Gender Identity Development Service, n.d.).

We have found that adult gender transition can be a complex and challenging process full of high expectations and deep frustration for the individual. This is exacerbated due to the time required to complete the gender transition pathway and the increasing difficulty for the National Health Service in the UK and other health services around the world to meet expectations and demand. We have witnessed anger and a deterioration in mental health status due to the long wait before entering the gender reassignment pathway, linked to a strong belief that life will be transformed for the better following transition accompanied by a real sense of urgency to achieve this. In reality, an improved life experience over the longer term, although enjoyed by many, cannot be guaranteed for all. An initial therapeutic exploration and understanding of personal development from early life and relationships can really help to prepare an individual for a journey that has the potential to improve their physical, emotional and mental health.

Parents, partners, relatives, colleagues, friends and employers also need to make significant transitions to adapt to a gender identity change. We have found that this can be particularly difficult for very close family and friends, who feel the loss of the gendered person they have known for many years (see Jackie and Ichika's, Richard's and Amy's case studies in Chapter 6). Some people transition fully and lead productive lives, whereas others transition only partially out of choice and feel content with this. However, after the initial excitement and relief of changing physically, a small number may wish to transition back to their original gender identity on account of reduced wellbeing or changes in life circumstances. This can cause serious surgical complications.

This introductory clarification of terms, ideas and concepts will make more sense as you read on. The debates around certain terminologies are sure to continue. We now begin to evidence our approach with a series of case studies from our clinical practice at various stages of the lifespan, beginning with first relationships. As we explained in the Preface, we have done our utmost to preserve the anonymity of these individuals from whom we have learned so much. The following chapters highlight sexual changes and challenges throughout the lifespan – from conception and birth to older age. We use our Reflect and Respond model to share our personal learning and development. Our material illustrates how this co-created intervention can be highly effective as we lay bare a deeply personal subject that so often remains unspoken, unaddressed and unresolved.

References

American Psychiatric Association (2013) *Diagnostic and statistical manual of mental disorders* (DSM-5) (5th edn). Arlington, VA: American Psychiatric Publishing.

Balint, M. (1964) *The doctor, his patient and the illness* (2nd edn). London: Pitman Medical.

Balint, M. and Balint, E. (1961) *Psychotherapeutic techniques in medicine*. London: Tavistock.

Batty, D. (2004) Mistaken identity. *Guardian*, 31 July. Available from: www.theguardian.com/society/2004/jul/31/health.socialcare (site accessed 23/11/2020).

Bond, T. and Holland, S. (1998) *The skills of clinical supervision for nurses*. Buckingham: Open University Press.

Burridge, S.M. (2017) Psychosexual counselling in an NHS setting. *Healthcare Counselling and Psychotherapy*, April, pp.14–17.

Centre for Suicide Prevention (n.d.) Transgender people and suicide. Available from: www.suicideinfo.ca/resource/transgender-people-suicide/ (site accessed 23/11/2020).

Etherington, K. (2004) *Becoming a reflexive researcher*. London: Jessica Kingsley.

Gender Identity Clinic (n.d.) Supporting patients waiting to be seen at GIC. Available from: https://gic.nhs.uk/gp-support/supporting-patients-waiting-seen-gender-identity-clinic/ (site accessed 21/11/2020).

Gender Identity Development Service (n.d.) Young people. Available from: https://gids.nhs.uk/young-people/ (site accessed 21/11/2020).

Gurney, K. (2020) *Mind the gap*. London: Headline.

Haas, A.P., Eliason, M., Mays, V. ... Clayton, P.J. (2011) Suicide and suicide risk in lesbian, gay, bisexual, and transgender populations: review and recommendations, *Journal of Homosexuality*, 58(1), pp. 10–51.

Hall, P. (2013) *Understanding and treating sex addiction*. London: Routledge.

Heath, H. and White, I. (2002) *The challenge of sexuality in health care*. Oxford: Blackwell Science Ltd.

Hellhammer, D.H. and Hellhammer, J. (eds) (2008) *Stress and the body–brain connection*. Basel: Karger.

Irwin, R. (2011) Recalling the early years of psychosexual nursing. Oral History, Spring, pp. 43–51.

Main, T. (1989) *The ailment and other psychoanalytic essays*. London: Free Association Books.

Malan, D.H. (1976) *The frontier of brief psychotherapy*. New York: Plenum Medical Book Company.

McNeil, J., Ellis, S.J. and Eccles, F.J.R. (2017). Suicide in trans populations: a systematic review of prevalence and correlates. *Psychology of Sexual Orientation and Gender Diversity*, 4(3), pp. 341–353.

Merriam-Webster (n.d.) Asexual. Available from: www.merriam-webster.com/dictionary/asexual (site accessed 23/11/2020).

Moore, A. (2009) Testicular cancer. *British Journal of Nursing*, 18(9), pp. 1182–1186.

Nagoski, E. (2015) *Come as you are*. London: Scribe.

Nimnuan, C., Hotopf, M. and Wessely, S. (2001) Medically unexplained symptoms: an epidemiological study in seven specialities. *Journal of Psychosomatic Research*, 51, pp. 361–367.

Penman, J.S. (1998) Action Research in the care of patients with sexual anxieties. *Nursing Standard*, 13(13–15), pp. 47–50.

Penman, J.S. (2009) Audit and evaluation of a psychosexual counselling service: identifying areas for development from a user-focused perspective. *Sexual and Relationship Therapy*, 24(3–4), pp. 347–367.

Penman, J.S. (2015) Engaging with persistent medically unexplained physical symptoms in healthcare. Doctoral Thesis, University of Bedfordshire. Available from: https://uobrep.openrepository.com/handle/10547/622044 (site accessed 28/01/2021).

Penman, J.S. (2018) Crossing the physical and mental health divide in partnership with 'hard to treat' patients with medically unresolved physical symptoms: from problem to solution. Version 4, December. Available from: www.researchgate.net/publication/321492531 (site accessed 28/01/2021).

Penman, J.S. (2019) Crossing the divide between physical and mental health interventions: a literature synthesis of interventions for medically unresolved persistent physical symptoms by evaluation research. Available from: www.researchgate.net/publication/332303578 (site accessed 28/01/2021).

Penman, J.S., Cook, E. and Randhawa, G. (2020) A collaborative brief engagement with medically unexplained sexual and other persistent physical symptoms: a realist service evaluation. *Sexual and Relationship Therapy*, 35(4). Available from: www.tandfonline.com/doi/abs/10.1080/14681994.2020.1736405 (site accessed 28/01/2021).

Rani, S. (2009) Menopause. *British Journal of Nursing*, 18(6), pp. 370–375.

Schön, D. (1983) *The reflective practitioner: how professionals think in action*. London: Temple Smith.

Schwandt, T.A. (2002) *Evaluation practice considered*. New York: Peter Lang.

Sharpe, M. (2013) Somatic symptoms: beyond 'medically unexplained'. *British Journal of Psychiatry*, 203, pp. 320–321.

Skrine, R. (1997) *Blocks and freedoms in sexual life*, Oxford: Radcliffe.

Tonelli, M.R. (2001) The limits of evidence-based medicine. *Respiratory Care*, 46(12), pp. 1435–1440.

Valins, L. (1992) *When a woman's body says no to sex: understanding and overcoming vaginismus*. London: Penguin.

Watkins, A. (ed.) (1997) *Mind–body medicine: a clinician's guide to psychoneuroimmunology*. Edinburgh: Churchill Livingstone.

Wells, D. (ed.) (2000). *Caring for sexuality in health and illness*. London: Churchill Livingstone.

WHO (n.d.) ICD-11 revision process. Available from: www.who.int/standards/classifications/classification-of-diseases/groups-that-were-involved-in-icd-11-revision-process (site accessed 26/11/2020).

WHO Regional Office for Europe (n.d.) WHO/Europe brief – transgender health in the context of ICD 11. Available from: www.euro.who.int/en/health-topics/health-determinants/gender/gender-definitions/whoeurope-brief-transgender-health-in-the-context-of-icd-11 (site accessed 26/11/2020).

Yüksel, S., Aslantas Ertekin, A., Ozturk, M., Bikmaz, P.S. and Oglagu, Z. (2017) A clinically neglected topic: risk of suicide in transgender individuals. *Archives of Neuropsychiatry*, 54(1), pp. 28–32.

1 Experiences in early years

First relationships and early sexual development

The mother-and-baby relationship represents the first relationship in the lifespan, beginning in utero or through the anticipation of arrival. Subsequently, the holding and eye-to-eye contact during the feeding process with the primary carer(s) facilitates falling in love with the infant through the release of the hormone oxytocin. Anxiety over feeding may temporarily affect bonding within the first intimate relationship. As the mother or primary carer breast or bottle feeds their child, this represents a good enough source of comfort, nourishment and physical acceptance to build the bond over time. Sexual development begins from birth with the baby's exploration of their own body and what may feel good and comforting. Toddlers' interest in their own and others' bodies can be an embarrassment but it is important for the parents, carers and HPs to find out which behaviours are age appropriate for sexual development. Professional guidelines are available online, such as the Brook 'Traffic Light Tool' (Brook, n.d.)

'Falling in love' with a father figure is just as important in the sexual development of a child. As the father connects emotionally with the infant, the child in turn learns the value of a different kind of relationship.

Affirmation provides a foundation from which the child can grow, giving security, a different type of play and discipline, and eventually the confidence to make friendships outside the family.

We acknowledge that parenting today takes many different forms that provide equal opportunity for the early development of intimate relationships.

During childhood there will also be many other relationships that will subtly or overtly influence sexual development, such as those with other adults, siblings, friends and teachers.

Influences on sexual development

In healthcare settings it is important to be aware of healthy sexual development and when safeguarding processes need to be initiated. There are powerful influences in society that impact on children as they grow up, which convey conflicting messages about the value of gender, body image and relationships, communicated through social media. Messages concerning sexual behaviour may conflict with the beliefs and attitudes of parents, families, schools, cultural and religious communities, leading to confusion and self-doubt in young people. Confusion and distress can be magnified among those who are questioning their gender identity and sexuality. National directives and sexual health messages, which tend to focus on rising sexually transmitted infections and teenage pregnancy rates, give the impression that all young people are sexually active. The combination of all these factors can become a source of internal compulsion and external coercion to become sexually active. Girls and boys talk about the immense pressure from their peers to have their first sexual experience. In contrast to the media's idealisation of sexual freedom, the young person with a number of sexual experiences is often labelled in derogatory terms by their peers, which can have negative consequences on their ongoing sexual development.

CELINE: AM I NORMAL?

A bright young girl, Celine, aged 16, went to see her GP for help with her low mood as this was affecting her school work. The GP listened carefully and asked her if there was anything she was worried about. She spoke about her fear that she wasn't normal; she didn't feel anything during occasional sex with an older boyfriend. The GP asked her to say a little more about what was really bothering her. Celine described how she hated her peer group criticising and judging others' sexual behaviours or, equally, ridiculing their choice not to have sex. Celine's understanding through listening to friends was that she should enjoy sex 'whatever' the circumstances. Because of this, Celine was concerned to find out if her lack of feeling during sex was normal. The GP discovered that Celine didn't really like her boyfriend. They came to agree that as Celine developed a trusting and respectful relationship in the future, sex was more likely to become a pleasure for her.

REFLECT

A lack of experience of rewarding relationships can lead to unrealistic expectations developed through the use of social media and peer pressure. As with Celine, this may lead to the belief that something is seriously wrong, causing considerable anxiety.

RESPOND

It may help to take an interest in the young person's perspective on the sexual difficulty before offering any reassurance or treatment.

Disruption to sexual development

Challenging life events during childhood, such as acrimonious divorce or the early death of a parent, may appear to be overcome at the time. However, as we hear from people about their sexual difficulties, an exploration of the cause often leads us back to significant experiences and relationships in early years. Subsequently, these experiences are found to impact on adult sexual relationships, presenting blocks to emotional and sexual intimacy and function. We have found that if changes in adult sexual experience are not due to a medical cause or medication, they are likely to have been triggered by a recent life event and later found linked to an early life experience.

Experiences of loss are very personal and can manifest in different ways.

The following two cases illustrate the unpredictable effects of loss in early life and the unexpected long-term effects on sexual intimacy.

AMANDA'S DISCONNECTION

A 36-year-old businesswoman, Amanda, was referred to a psychosexual therapy clinic complaining of complete loss of sexual desire within two successive same-sex relationships. Having initially enjoyed sex with each partner, there was no obvious explanation for her lack of feelings. Amanda was also adamant that she did not want children. The therapist reflected with Amanda on her early years to explore any predisposing or precipitating factors. Showing little emotion, Amanda described how her unemotional parents had separated when she was eight years old and how confusing and disruptive this had been for her. She was given no opportunity to talk about her difficult feelings. Amanda and the therapist discovered that she had learned to block out her feelings as way of coping as a child. Her partner would do everything she could to arouse her but she remained emotionally and physically disconnected. Despite a good deal of resistance, in time Amanda acknowledged her anger with her parents and her own fear of separation in long-term relationships. Once her anger and fear were recognised, this seemed to allow Amanda to talk to her partner and reconnect emotionally. After this she reported a reawakening of a pleasurable response to physical intimacy.

BEN'S BURIED LOSS

Ben, a young man in his late twenties with a long-term partner and child, presented for general counselling for intermittent low mood over many years. He described how masturbation to images of women on the internet provided relief from stress. The counsellor asked about his current sexual relationship. Ben explained that he avoided sex although he loved his long-term girlfriend, Jessica, very much. They had discussed the sexual difficulty together and felt their problems were due to Ben's use of pornography.

During their frequent arguments, whenever Jessica cried, Ben described feelings of deep distress and impotence. When the therapist asked if he had ever felt like this before, after a moment of thought Ben recalled an incident that had happened when he was four years old. He talked of hearing an agonising scream when his mother discovered the lifeless body of his baby sister. She was inconsolable. Following this event, despite his four-year-old's efforts to make her feel better, he did not succeed. His mother was so wrapped up in her grief that she was unable to notice or respond to him. In his current relationship Ben made every effort to be a helpful partner and dad, despite continuing to feel a deep sense of loneliness. During the course of his therapy, he recognised that this awful feeling of impotence was relieved momentarily by masturbating to sexual images and this means of finding comfort and control had subsequently diverted his sexual attention away from Jessica. But more than this, he realised that his mother's rejection of him

> was now playing out within his own intimate relationship: Ben was rejecting Jessica without knowing it. Over a period of time, having recognised this pattern, Ben was able to initiate enjoyable sex with Jessica and his compulsion to masturbate using pornography for relief and comfort was significantly reduced.

REFLECT

The consequence of unexpressed emotion can have a powerful effect throughout life and within intimate relationships. The details of Amanda's and Ben's presentations illustrate the negative impact of previously buried memories of earlier life experiences and their potential effects on intimacy in adult life (see Jamie's case study in Chapter 3).

RESPOND

Asking about early life relationships can often open up important connections to current difficulties.

Childhood sexual abuse

Childhood sexual abuse (CSA) and sexual exploitation is a sad and complex reality for many and can have a lifelong effect on sexual health and wellbeing. Through our practice, we have often observed patients internalising rage and resentment towards family members and significant adults whom they feel should have prevented or stopped it, resulting in low self-esteem and other mental health difficulties. Walker argues, 'Anger towards the abuser and often also towards those adults who did not prevent it can persist either consciously or unconsciously, when it may be turned against the self and incorporated into self-loathing' (Walker, 2001: p. 85).

As well as mental health and emotional difficulties, we have found a variety of persistent physical symptoms which may be linked to unspoken pain and sexual trauma: palpitations, shortness of breath, chest, abdominal, genital and pelvic pain, skin conditions and frequent headaches are only some of many examples. All these require medical attention when discovered through the psychosexual consultation. The Patient Health Questionnaire Somatic Symptom Severity (PHQ-15) can help to reveal the physical burden and what can be done about it through further discussion (Kroenke, Spitzer and Williams, 2002).

An HP who observes signs of physical distress and listens without judgement may allow for an important disclosure (see Figure 0.3 in the Introduction). This brief cooperative rapport can be instrumental in supporting the patient to begin the journey of recovery. Although the disclosure may bring back painful memories, the non-judgemental approach of the HP will bring relief and confidence to the patient to break their silence and then move forward. Local safeguarding procedures (for both child and adult) must be followed at all times for their own and others' protection (UK Home Office, 2018).

The ramifications of sexual abuse can also have a profoundly disturbing effect on the family and wider community. Individuals are often reluctant to disclose abuse for fear of further harm and the judgement of others. Through a qualitative evaluation of a psychosexual intervention, a cycle of common factors were found to delay the recovery of medically unresolved physical symptoms (see Figure 1.1).

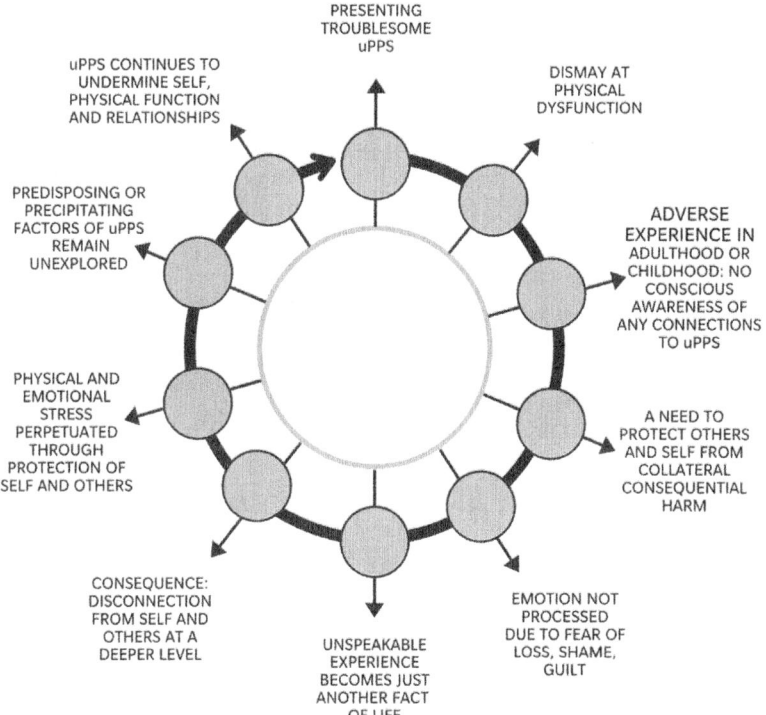

Figure 1.1 The cycle of unresolved persistent physical symptoms (uPPS). Source: Penman, 2015.

On many occasions we have observed ongoing emotional hurt and physical pain when childhood sexual abuse or sexual exploitation remains an unspeakable, well-guarded secret.

> **LINDA: MUMMIES DON'T CRY**
>
> Linda, aged 45, was seen by her GP for ongoing depression and irritable bowel syndrome (IBS). She revealed that she had been sexually abused by a close family member from her earliest childhood memory. During the abuse she learned to shut down her feelings to survive. As a result of this, in adulthood she struggled to show any emotion towards her family. Recently, following a family bereavement, her distressed 8-year-old daughter asked her, 'Mummies don't cry, do they?' This comment deeply shocked and upset Linda and triggered her search for help.

REFLECT

It is not only memories that can be locked away, but powerful feelings too. Linda's daughter seems to have understood from being close to her mum that mothers just don't allow sadness and tears to show. She may carry this into her own adult life.

RESPOND

By registering the emotional aspect of what is said, we can understand so much more readily what is causing pain and how failing to talk about it can impact not only on health and wellbeing but also on those who are closest to us.

> **ELSIE'S CARE OF HER MOTHER**
>
> A heavily pregnant HP undertook a home visit to assess 79-year-old Elsie's numerous medically unresolved symptoms. Unexpectedly, on seeing that the HP was heavily pregnant, Elsie, through angry tears, revealed her past sexual abuse for the first time in her life. Realising

> the importance of this moment, with empathy, the HP encouraged her to tell her more. Elsie disclosed that during her teenage years she was forced to have sex with her step-father; if she refused, he threatened to have sex with other women outside her parents' marriage. Elsie knew this would devastate her mother and she felt she must protect her. In that moment, the HP felt Elsie's conflict and pain as if it were yesterday. As Elsie wept, she revealed that during this time she had become pregnant by her step-father and had lost the baby through miscarriage. Her expression of grief was profound as she recognised that since that time she had never been able to enjoy sex. On the next contact with her, Elsie described how her weeping had continued through the night but now, a couple of weeks later, she was feeling so much lighter and her physical pain was much improved.

REFLECT

There had been no safe place for Elsie to express her anger, loss and hurt as a child or adult for fear of causing further harm to herself and others which she could not bear. It seems it is never too late to speak out, be listened to and believed, or to facilitate the disclosure of previously unspeakable events, even though the teller and the listener may both feel vulnerable.

RESPOND

If we allow ourselves not only to ask but also to hear and acknowledge what is said, this can be an opening for beneficial outcomes.

Elsie and Linda are examples of the lifelong impact of childhood sexual abuse within the family, diminishing their natural emotional responses and often leading to physical distress. Furthermore, in cases of child sexual exploitation the young person is socialised into believing it is acceptable and then becomes caught in a cycle of self-harming behaviours, often causing unrecognised relationship, emotional and physical damage.

Child sexual exploitation

There has been significant multi-agency awareness-raising around the complex issue of child sexual exploitation (CSE) and organisations are getting better at identifying those at risk. However, due to the extensive grooming process, many young people do not recognise that they are being sexually exploited. The National Society for the Prevention of Cruelty to Children (NSPCC, n.d.) defines the problem as follows: 'Child sexual exploitation (CSE) is a type of sexual abuse. When a child or young person is exploited, they're given things, like gifts, drugs, money, status and affection, in exchange for performing sexual activities.'

The NSPCC confirms our findings in practice that children or young people may be deceived into believing they are in a loving, fun relationship. They may be given welcome attention, invited to parties and given drugs and alcohol, groomed and exploited online or ultimately trafficked within or across national borders for the purpose of sexual exploitation. CSE can also be part of meeting the sexual expectations within youth gang culture and accepted as non-harmful by gang members. The phenomenon of drug trafficking across England, known as 'County Lines' (UK Home Office, 2018), often includes the sexual exploitation of young people. The complexities relating to coercion by threats, money, drugs and alcohol is highly likely to disrupt and undermine a person's identity and ongoing sexual development.

Jade's case shows that sexual exploitation can happen within a family.

JADE'S STRUGGLE

Jade, now 25 years old, was introduced to recreational drugs by an older male relative at the age of ten. The perpetrator went on to use her drug dependency as a way of eliciting sexual acts from her, so that she could 'earn' the money to pay for her habit. Over the years, Jade became known to the police for her angry outbursts and her verbal abuse of others. Subsequently she made every effort to make a life for herself and her daughter, but when things went wrong, she became overwhelmed with feelings of hopelessness and at these times was unable to meet her daughter's emotional needs. Feeling a failure and seeking companionship through old 'friends', she found herself falling back into drugs and alcohol misuse as a way of surviving. This cycle of abuse seriously affected her ability to form and sustain any relationship that did not include drugs, let alone a healthy sexual relationship in adulthood.

Experiences in early years 29

REFLECT

Jade's story illustrates the importance of a non-judgemental interpretation of destructive behaviours which may be indicative of anger and frustration at not being heard.

RESPOND

In complex cases such as Jade's, instead of being critical of her outbursts, it may help to look behind the behaviour to identify the root cause.

JAZ: KEEPING HERSELF SAFE?

A 14-year-old girl, Jaz, had an appointment booked for a full sexual health screen and contraceptive implant. On arrival she was accompanied by a support worker who informed the nurse that Jaz was living in a local residential home, having been removed from a child sexual exploitation situation. The support worker, with Jaz's consent, offered the telephone number of the residential home and a password in order for the nurse to gain further information. Jaz was then given the opportunity to come into the consultation room on her own, but she insisted she wanted the support worker with her.

On discussion to assess her risk of contracting a sexually transmitted infection (STI) and contraception needs, Jaz gave no indication that she had been at risk. Although the support worker remained silent, the nurse noted body language that indicated that Jaz wasn't revealing the true extent of the sexual risks she had been taking. Jaz agreed to a full sexual health screen but refused to let the nurse proceed with the contraceptive implant. An arrangement was made for her to return to the clinic at a later date. The nurse could only hope that she would do so.

REFLECT

Without the information provided by the support worker, the nurse would not have appreciated how vulnerable Jaz was, as she was unaware of the risks associated with her sexual activity. There is evidence that many victims of CSE do not consider themselves 'victims' (UK Home Office, 2018).

RESPOND

Sexual history taking can be helpfully supported by an HP's awareness of personal context, body language, place of living, use of words and attitude. Sexual history taking holds the key to the practice of sexual health medicine. It provides the basis for treatment, prevention, education and sexual health promotion. The most important aspect of taking a sexual history lies in the concept that the patient needs to be reassured that their privacy and confidentiality are paramount. It is essential to ensure that the conversation is not overheard or interrupted.

> Only experience and skill in taking a sexual history can sympathetically encourage patients to reveal the intimate details of their private life that are necessary to determine the choice of examination, laboratory investigations, diagnosis, follow up and, in particular, contact tracing. All information sought should be justifiable on one or other of these grounds. In some cases, it is often helpful to be explicit about these reasons, to allay the patient's fear or embarrassment evoked by these questions.
>
> (Jones and Barton, 2004: pp. 444–446)

CHLOE'S NORMAL

At 17, Chloe was referred for psychosexual counselling by the local community mental health team, who requested support in relation to her current sexual relationship and the impact of recent experiences of sexual exploitation. With her parents' consent, Chloe was placed in care for nine months in order to escape from a so-called child sexual exploitation network. Chloe was unable to recognise how the group of older boys whom she and her girlfriends considered friends were sexually grooming and exploiting them. The sexual acts they were asked to perform were 'just what we did … it was normal'.

After many worrying incidents which caused her parents serious concern, they told their local Social Services that they were unable to convince Chloe of the risks she was taking or protect her. Chloe was taken into care several counties away. On returning home during the early stages of therapy, she was able to share how much shame and guilt she felt for her own actions, having realised how much her behaviour had distressed her parents. This hurt her badly and was her greatest regret. Furthermore, Chloe was unspeakably angry and upset that her girlfriends had not protected her when she was singled out one night for a specific sexual assault. One had even recorded the incident, laughing. Chloe felt this was something for which she could never forgive her. Curiously, though, there was little expression of anger towards the gang of boys, some of whom were 'nicer' than others.

Chloe gets angry with her new boyfriend, they have rows, he drinks to cope with their fallouts, she feels she is making all the effort, he controls where she goes, she knows they are not good for each other, but she feels that she could not survive without him at the moment.

REFLECT

While Chloe refused to acknowledge the harm inflicted by her 'friendships', she did acknowledge how important these were to her sense of wellbeing at the time. She struggled to accept that her anger at her current boyfriend may have belonged somewhere else. It will be some time before she understands that she could survive without a less than healthy relationship. Non-judgemental health and social care workers were her lifeline for her survival.

RESPOND

Trust and confidence can be built over time by understanding the young person's viewpoint from the outset. Supporting recovery from the effects of CSE will need to continue into future adult relationships.

Female genital mutilation

Female genital mutilation (FGM) includes all procedures involving the partial or total removal of the external female genitalia or any other injury to female genital organs for non-medical reasons. FGM is also known as female circumcision or cutting, and by other terms, such as sunna, gudniin, halalays, tahur, megrez and khitan. It is usually carried out on young girls between infancy and the age of 15, most commonly before puberty starts. Four main types of FGM have been described:

- Type 1 (clitoridectomy) – removing part or all of the clitoris
- Type 2 (excision) – removing part or all of the clitoris and the inner labia (the lips that surround the vagina), with or without removal of the labia majora (the larger outer lips)
- Type 3 (infibulation) – narrowing the vaginal opening by creating a seal, formed by cutting and repositioning the labia
- Type 4 – other harmful procedures to the female genitals, including pricking, piercing, cutting, scraping or burning the area

(World Health Organisation, n.d.)

FGM is practised for a variety of complex reasons, usually in the belief that it is beneficial for the girl. It has no health benefits; rather, it harms girls and women in many ways. FGM is a human rights violation and a form of child abuse, breaching the United Nations Convention on the Rights of the Child, amounting to a severe form of violence against women and girls (End FGM European Network, 2016). There are many physical and emotional complications affecting survival and dignity that may remain unacknowledged in communities that practise FGM. However, many young girls remain at risk of 'cutting' due to the belief that this makes them acceptable for marriage.

FURAH IN PAIN

Furah, a 20-year-old woman, attended a contraceptive and sexual health clinic. She had recently married but disclosed that the marriage had not been consummated due to her experiencing excruciating pain when she and her husband attempted sex. She had a vaginal discharge which she thought could be the cause and wanted to get it treated as the couple were planning to try for a baby.

After having swabs taken by the doctor she was referred to the sexual health advisor (SHA) as the doctor had observed that she had been a victim of Type 3 FGM – infibulation. The doctor whispered this information to the SHA as he ushered Furah into the SHA's consultation room. The SHA felt at a disadvantage as she had not seen the genitals for herself, yet she was expected to raise the issue with Furah. The SHA carefully asked Furah if she had had any changes/operations on her genital area in the past. She said no, looked confused and seemed not to know what the SHA was talking about.

The SHA realised Furah had no idea (or had blocked out any memory) of what may have been done to her, but she needed to know what had been seen during the doctor's examination and how this may impact on her becoming pregnant.

The SHA gave Furah a mirror to look at her genital area in privacy. A chaperone was offered but declined, and the SHA took time to explain some of the changes that had been made to Furah's vulval area, probably when she was a young girl. They were then able to discuss the benefits of a surgical referral for deinfibulation in order to facilitate more comfortable sex and increase the feasibility of a vaginal delivery if pregnancy were achieved in the future.

DR TANOUS: WRAPPED UP

The health visitor (HV) made a home visit to a newly arrived immigrant couple – Mr and Dr Tanous – in order to introduce them to the local healthcare system and enquire about any health needs. The wife spoke English with ease and was already professionally employed. She told the HV that her husband was not at home but reported they were settling in well and were hoping to start a family in the New Year. The HV asked whether she had any questions about pregnancy. Dr Tanous started to say that it had been suggested on examination by her GP for vaginal discharge that a small surgical procedure may be required to open her up as she had been subjected to female circumcision as a child. Dr Tanous was aware of her cutting at the age of eight but was still outraged by this suggestion. The HV discovered that, for this woman, 'opening her up' would make her feel dirty, ashamed and sexually undesirable to her husband. Therefore, it was out of the question. The HV did not address this further at the time but at a subsequent visit she was able to explain, particularly in view of a possible pregnancy, that the corrective surgery could be beneficial in reducing delivery complications.

REFLECT

In both cases the HPs faced unexpectedly challenging consultations. The HV was initially taken aback by Dr Tanous' defensive response but began to understand a little more about the historical social imperative in some cultures for FGM to make young girls acceptable for marriage.

RESPOND

All professionals need to respond to local guidelines during discussions with colleagues, especially if there are younger girls within the family who may be at risk. It is helpful, as always, to show respect, kindness and transparency to the individual in order to understand their perspectives prior to explaining the legal position (GOV.UK, n.d.).

FGM is now recognised harmful to the woman as it has the potential to cause physical and emotional wounds, and it is illegal in the UK. The practice is known to decrease sexual pleasure and can become the cause of serious genitourinary complications.

References

Brook (n.d.) Sexual behaviours traffic light tool. Available from: https://legacy.brook.org.uk/brook_tools/traffic/Brook_Traffic_Light_Tool.pdf (site accessed 23/11/2020).

End FGM European Network (2016) UN Convention on the Rights of the Child. Available from: www.endfgm.eu/resources/international/un-convention-on-the-rights-of-the-child/ (site accessed 23/11/2020).

GOV.UK (n.d.) Female genital mutilation: resource pack. Available from: www.gov.uk/government/publications/female-genital-mutilation-resource-pack/female-genital-mutilation-resource-pack (site accessed 23/11/2020).

Jones, R. and Barton, S. (2004) Introduction to history taking and principles of sexual health. *Postgraduate Medical Journal*, 80, pp. 444–446.

Kroenke, K., Spitzer, R.L. and Williams, J.B.W. (2002) The PHQ-15: validity of a new measure for evaluating somatic symptom severity. *Psychosomatic Medicine*, 64, pp. 258–266.

NSPCC (n.d.) Child sexual exploitation. Available from: www.nspcc.org.uk/what-is-child-abuse/types-of-abuse/child-sexual-exploitation/ (site accessed 23/11/2020).

Penman, J.S. (2015) Engaging with persistent medically unexplained physical symptoms in healthcare. Doctoral thesis, University of Bedfordshire. Available from: https://uobrep.openrepository.com/handle/10547/622044 (site accessed 28/01/2021).

UK Home Office (2018) *Criminal exploitation of children and vulnerable adults: county lines guidance*. Available from: https://assets.publishing.service.gov.uk/

government/uploads/system/uploads/attachment_data/file/863323/HOCount yLinesGuidance_-_Sept2018.pdf (site accessed 29/01/2021).

Walker, S. (2001) The relevance of past history, in R. Skrine and H. Montford (eds), *Psychosexual medicine: an introduction*. London: Arnold.

World Health Organisation (n.d.) Female genital mutilation. Available from: www.who.int/en/news-room/fact-sheets/detail/female-genital-mutilation (site accessed 23/11/2020).

Further reading

Casey, L. (2015). *Reflections on child sexual exploitation*. Available from: https://assets.publishing.service.gov.uk/government/uploads/system/uploads/attachment_data/file/418394/Louise_Casey_report_into_CSE_template_format__4_.pdf (site accessed 23/11/2020).

Crown Prosecution Service (2019) *Prostitution and exploitation of prostitution*. Available from: www.cps.gov.uk/legal-guidance/prostitution-and-exploitation-prostitution (site accessed 21/11/2020).

National Crime Agency (n.d.) Available from: www.nationalcrimeagency.gov.uk (site accessed 23/11/2020).

NHS (n.d.) National FGM support clinics. Available from: www.nhs.uk/conditions/female-genital-mutilation-fgm/national-fgm-support-clinics/ (site accessed 21/11/2020).

NSPCC Learning (n.d.) Safeguarding children and child protection. Available from: https://learning.nspcc.org.uk/safeguarding-child-protection/ (site accessed 23/11/2020).

Rethink Mental Illness (n.d.) Available from: https://rethink.org (site accessed 23/11/2020).

UNICEF (n.d.) How we protect children's rights with the UN Convention on the Rights of the Child. Available from: www.unicef.org.uk/what-we-do/un-convention-child-rights/ (site accessed 29/01/2021).

Contact details

NSPCC: 0800 028 3550 or fgmhelp@nspcc.org.uk.

2 Reproductive years

Teenage pregnancy

Teenage conception can be viewed in many different ways. As with pregnancies in general, a teenage pregnancy can be planned or unplanned, and it is not necessarily a negative event. The desire for a pregnancy in early teenage years has sometimes been associated with low aspirations, poverty and intergenerational patterns. The absence of healthy family attachments and the need to be needed can be driving factors for a young girl to have her own baby. Whilst teenage pregnancy may be a subject of controversy, in some societies early motherhood is the norm and a source of family pride.

Alison Hadley, Director of the Teenage Pregnancy Knowledge Exchange, has written extensively on the need for all children and young people to receive high-quality sex and relationship education (SRE) as well as easy access to contraception and sexual health services (see Hadley, 2017; Hadley, Chandra and Ingham, 2016; see also FSRH, 2020). School nurses may need to provide extra help for young people with known risk factors for early pregnancy, such as frequent absences from school. Guidance for healthy sex and relationship educators in schools to identify and support young people experiencing or at risk of CSE, linked with prevention of early pregnancy to enhance a young person's life chances, is readily available in the UK.

LUCY AND HER TWINS

Lucy, a 16-year-old only child who found herself 22 weeks pregnant with twins, attended an antenatal clinic with her mother and her 17-year-old boyfriend. The midwife asked how she would cope with the arrival of two babies. Lucy replied that she had already started to attend parentcraft classes and had offered to help out at a nursery in order to gain experience in how to care for her babies. With the confidence to seek out information that would help her, together with the support of her mother, boyfriend and his parents, the midwife saw that the pregnancy was developing into a positive experience for Lucy, her babies and her extended family.

REFLECT

Teenage pregnancies can present in different ways. We often make early assumptions about young people's coping skills which can trigger anxiety and concern in the HP. This may blind us to the reality of the situation.

RESPOND

Being open to take in the details and clues provided can allow professional advice to be adapted to the personal circumstances, which in turn allows everyone to feel happier with the consultation outcome.

VICKY'S SURPRISE

Vicky, aged 15, dressed in her school uniform, arrived at her local Accident & Emergency department with her mother, suffering acute abdominal pain. She was referred to the antenatal ward with a full-term pregnancy in early onset of labour. Vicky had not disclosed the pregnancy to anyone, including her mother, who was a single parent of three daughters. Within 24 hours the baby was born. During this time Vicky's mother experienced shock, anger, concern and finally relief once the baby was safely delivered. Vicky revealed that she had had sex just once with a local boy whilst on holiday. The next day the midwife observed Vicky quietly breastfeeding her baby boy, surrounded by her adoring mother and sisters. The mother turned to the midwife and said, 'We went on holiday last summer and look what we came home with – our very own Italian stallion!'

REFLECT

See 'Lucy and her twins', above.

RESPOND

Hearing and seeing the reality of the situation from the person's lived perspective can be a relief and a cause for shared celebration. In Vicky's and Lucy's stories there are similarities of emotional expression: shock and concern developed into intimacy and attachment between mother and baby and their family. However, there can be difficulties with bonding and attachment if the young person has further demands placed upon her.

AVA'S NEED

Ava, a young mother, came into the pregnancy dating scan room with her sleeping ten-month-old son in a pushchair. Before Ava got on the couch for the scan, she suddenly shouted at the child to wake up and look at his brother or sister on the screen. He began to wail, which irritated her. The HP was very concerned about Ava's unrealistic expectation of her child and the subsequent demands that a new-born baby would bring. There was a brief discussion about the pressures of another baby and the HP asked if she would like further support. With Ava's consent, the HP subsequently made contact with the midwife, suggesting a referral to a local family support centre where Ava could attend parenting classes and receive care for herself and her toddler before the new baby arrived.

REFLECT

In this instance, the HP shows that witnessing and merely noting a possible risk of harm, even within a brief consultation, is not enough. This, we find, also relates to any kind of response that we might make when we witness potential harm to another. In Ava's case, acting on it in the moment of the consultation with honesty and respect simplified the situation. An agreed, non-judgemental referral back to the midwife ensured the possibility of multi-disciplinary support for the mother before the stress of another baby overwhelmed her care of her toddler.

RESPOND

In challenging situations there may be ethical issues to address before taking action. How often do we see something of concern, walk on by and imagine that it is someone else's responsibility? Early intervention may prevent future difficulties between the adult and the child.

Young mothers may need additional support during the postnatal period to access effective contraceptive care. The majority of the adult population of England are sexually active and need signposting to quality sexual health services in order to improve health and wellbeing.

Contraceptive provision

The introduction of integrated contraception and sexual health services (CASH) was intended to offer easier access and information to local residents. Currently, the UK's local authorities commission comprehensive open-access sexual health services, including free STI testing and treatment, notification of the sexual partners of infected persons and free provision of contraception (FSRH, 2020). Some specialised services are directly commissioned by clinical commissioning groups (CCGs), and at the national level by NHS England (GOV.UK, 2013).

A person's first sexual experience may have a profound effect on future sexual function even if the two are not consciously linked. The first contact in seeking advice and help regarding contraception and sexual health can also have a significant impact on sexual confidence and function. The value of a welcoming environment for all, whether the young person attends in a group, with their parent, carer or partner, or on their own, cannot be overestimated. A non-judgemental and open approach allows those who may feel reluctant, embarrassed or shy to access contraceptive services and feel supported in making informed choices regarding their sexual health.

BLEEDING ANNA

Anna was aged 22 when she started to attend for contraceptive care on a regular basis, but she soon found problems with each method she was given. The clinic's staff became exasperated in their attempts to meet her needs and Anna never seemed satisfied. Eventually the nurse asked her thoughtfully, 'What's sex like for you at the moment?' After a moment Anna tearfully replied, 'I can't

> have sex because it's too painful!' In this admission the nurse caught a glimpse of Anna's problem and asked when the pain had first started. Anna said that her first sexual experience – about five years previously – had been very painful and she had bled afterwards. She also expressed her fear of this repeating. The memory of it was powerful enough to stop her from trying sexual intercourse again, leaving tension, pain and dissatisfaction.

REFLECT

The nurse was able to see beyond the shared exasperation and get a sense of the underlying cause of Anna's dissatisfaction. She asked Anna if she would like to be referred for psychosexual therapy to explore her fear and find a way to pain-free sex (see 'Professional training and support' in Chapter 13). Our findings are supported by two members of the Institute of Psychosexual Medicine UK, Montford and Skrine (1993), who suggest that women often blame their contraceptive method for physical symptoms that may be completely unrelated.

RESPOND

When nothing seems to help a frequent attender to resolve their problem, listen with an open mind to try to understand what is going on and why. Changing the contraceptive method might seem an easy option for both the patient and the HP, but it may be necessary to identify a completely different underlying reason for the dissatisfaction.

Heightened psychosexual awareness followed by the acquisition of enhanced HP skills can therefore be useful in brief interventions, as the following example demonstrates.

> ### TINA AND LEVI: DOUBLE DUTCH
>
> At 17 years old, Tina attended a clinic with her partner Levi to access oral contraception. They were offered condoms as a temporary back-up. Levi looked very uncomfortable and embarrassed and said that he didn't need them. The nurse gently asked why and with

a flushed face he replied that he had used a condom once before and it hadn't worked. She asked what he meant by this and Levi said, 'OK, after I put the condom on, I lost it.' The nurse explained that this is very common – both younger and older men often lose their erection in these circumstances. She suggested to the couple that they should experiment with the condom together as part of their sexual play or Levi could practise on his own to gain confidence.

REFLECT

This confident and calm brief intervention with Levi aptly illustrates how a sexual concern or loss of confidence can be addressed in the moment and prevented from becoming a long-term sexual dysfunction.

Of course, lack of contraceptive protection during heterosexual encounters may lead to conception.

RESPOND

Sometimes a simple, swift HP intervention can prevent an issue becoming an embarrassing, chronic problem.

Pregnancy

Pregnancy can be an emotive subject. The news of a positive pregnancy test can generate a surprising mix of emotions. Even a planned pregnancy can evoke feelings of joy, excitement, anticipation, fear or uncertainty in the woman and her partner. The news can also bring to life painful memories of previous loss or complications in pregnancy (Wells, 2000).

At the beginning of pregnancy many women experience a mixture of feelings at the prospect of carrying a child. This may also apply to pregnancies in same-sex relationships and surrogate mothers. The potential stress on both parties and their families should be kept in mind, and contact with the midwife can allow any concerns or difficulties to be aired and sensitively addressed (Stahl, 2020). Increasingly over the last two decades, many women in the West have focused on their careers and consequently have babies later in life. In contrast to teenage pregnancy, such pregnancies tend to generate minimal concern regarding the mother's ability to cope. However, this is challenged by Sandra and Adam's story.

SANDRA AND ADAM: OVER- AND UNDER-PREPARED

Sandra and Adam were in their forties and had recently had twin girls. They were both academics and had experienced a life of routine. In the months leading up to the births, Sandra had read every expert advice book on childbirth and baby care. Therefore, it was a surprise when they struggled to cope with simple tasks such as bathing and feeding in the immediate postnatal period. Sandra would write down a timetable for feeding the girls but as soon as one woke up earlier than expected, she would become upset, tearful and panicky. This reaction impacted on all around her, blocking her ability to bond with the babies and increasing her husband's anxiety. Both sets of grandparents were in their eighties and not well enough to provide the couple with practical support. Eventually, after 18 days of care and education by the maternity staff, they were encouraged to leave the hospital.

REFLECT

Sandra and Adam would have triggered few, if any, concerns during antenatal care. However, despite their intellectual ability and thorough preparation for the birth of their twins, their anxiety and feelings of loss of control blocked their ability to cope and subsequently bond with their babies. Their over-preparedness could have been masking deep-rooted fears and anxiety about the responsibility of becoming parents. Postnatal care is just as important to support new parents.

RESPOND

Is it possible to identify and support a couple or individual and address their anxiety earlier in the healthcare journey?

JOANNE: A RUINED MOMENT

At the age of 38, Joanne, a mother of six children, attended an antenatal clinic to confirm another pregnancy. Unexpectedly, the obstetrics and gynaecology (O&G) consultant ushered a tearful Joanne and her red-faced, angry husband into the midwife's room and left. Looking at Joanne's tear-stained face and furious partner, the midwife turned to the couple and asked, 'What on earth has happened?' Through her sobs, Joanne explained that once the pregnancy had been confirmed, the consultant had launched into a lecture about sterilisation.

Joanne went on to explain that this baby was a much-wanted addition to the family and that the doctor's assumption that they already had enough children had ruined what should have been a happy moment. Her husband angrily interjected that he provided well for his family and they were not reliant on state benefits. The midwife apologised for the incident and took the time to enquire about their growing family.

REFLECT

Joanne's story shows how the professional anxieties and assumptions of any HP may have unintended negative impacts. In our experience, the trauma of unhelpful words is rarely forgotten. In this instance, the midwife's investment of a small amount of time at a crucial point probably prevented a complaint and helped to restore the couple's 'happy moment'.

RESPOND

Personal awareness that professional anxieties and assumptions can have negative impacts on the individual prompts us to ask the individual or couple how they are experiencing their particular situation.

Another example follows.

HEATHER'S STEM DISTRACTION

Heather was contacted by the midwife to arrange an antenatal booking appointment. Heather had been avoiding making the appointment and sounded distracted during the telephone call, as if she were too busy to speak.

> On meeting Heather face to face, the midwife noticed that Heather was keen to get through the details and seemed eager to leave. This prompted the midwife to ask, 'How are you feeling about this pregnancy?' Heather visibly relaxed and tearfully confided to the midwife that she had become pregnant in order to use stem cells from the new baby's umbilical cord to facilitate her two-year-old daughter's treatment for leukaemia. She wanted to get back to the children's ward to be with her daughter as soon as she could. On leaving, Heather said to the midwife, 'You must think I'm awful.'

REFLECT

Unexpected reactions or behaviour, such as Heather's, may benefit from a moment of exploration which allows further understanding of context. Any form of unexpected behaviour may mask hidden difficulties.

RESPOND

Creating an opportunity for an individual to talk can offer immediate relief of personal distress and lessen fears. Asking what further help the individual needs can reveal a more appropriate pathway towards a better experience and improved wellbeing.

In our experience, sometimes the pressure to have a baby, whatever the cause, can be so immense that it leads to sexual difficulties. Heather had no desire for sex with her partner once she had conceived and this was adding to the couple's tension and worry. Whatever the circumstances, we have found that women value being asked about sex during pregnancy, and post-termination of pregnancy problems with sex may, for some, feel like punishments.

Termination of pregnancy

Some conditions lead to a medically recommended termination of pregnancy (TOP), whilst some people decide not to continue with a pregnancy for social and emotional reasons. TOP clinics are often very busy, and personal discomfort or time pressure may lead an HP to assume that someone else has already given the patient time to talk.

Terminating a pregnancy is a challenge for women and their HPs. It is a decision that has to be made under pressure within certain time limits and there can be lasting repercussions for the woman's and her partner's physical and emotional wellbeing (Skrine, 1997)

In our experience we can never know how a termination will impact on people's lives unless we take the time to listen and adapt our approach to each person. And it remains every woman's right to change her mind at any time, even after admission for a TOP.

During therapy, we have found the following psychosexual problems to be associated with termination of pregnancy:

- Loss of sexual desire
- Painful sex
- Loss of erections
- Guilt blocking feelings of sexual pleasure

EVE'S HIDDEN GRIEF

At 48 years old, Eve was referred by her GP for psychosexual therapy on account of loss of sexual desire. She was worried that the lack of intimacy was affecting her relationship with her husband. She talked proudly of her family, especially her two daughters, but briefly mentioned that she had had a TOP between her two girls. The counsellor asked her about this and Eve began to cry loudly and painfully. Both she and the counsellor were shocked and surprised by the depth of her response. Despite being advised to terminate the pregnancy due to a genetic abnormality and going through with it, the uncontrollable feeling of loss that poured out of Eve was overwhelming.

REFLECT

Eve's hidden loss was found to have significantly affected her sexual desire. After her grief was expressed and released, she noticed the return of her sexual desire.

RESPOND

Allowing the outpouring of grief, however noisy or uncomfortable this may be, can be valuable and often long overdue. There are a number of ways in which loss is experienced during the reproductive years by both men and women. We outline some of these in the next chapter.

References

Faculty of Sexual and Reproductive Healthcare (FSRH) (2020) Press releases and statements. Available from: www.fsrh.org/news/fsrh-statement-teenage-pregnancy-q2-2019/ (site accessed 23/11/2020).

GOV. UK (2013) Commissioning sexual health services and interventions: best practice guidance for local authorities. Available from: www.gov.uk/government/publications/commissioning-sexual-health-services-and-interventions-best-practice-guidance-for-local-authorities (site accessed 23/11/2020).

Hadley, A. (2017) *Teenage pregnancy and young parenthood (adolescence and society)*. Abingdon: Routledge.

Hadley, A., Chandra Mouli, V. and Ingham, R. (2016) Implementing the United Kingdom government's 10-year teenage pregnancy strategy for England (1999–2010): applicable lessons for other countries. *Journal of Adolescent Health*, 59(1), pp. 68–74.

Montford, H. and Skrine, R. (eds) (1993) *Contraceptive care: meeting individual needs*. London: Chapman and Hall.

Skrine, R. (1997) *Blocks and freedoms in sexual life*. Oxford: Radcliffe.

Stahl, A. (2020) New study: millennial women are delaying having children due to their careers. Available from: www.forbes.com/sites/ashleystahl/2020/05/01 (site accessed 29/01/2021).

Wells, D. (Ed.) (2000). *Caring for sexuality in health and illness*. London: Churchill Livingstone.

Further reading

National Institutes of Health (n.d.) Stem cell Information. Available from: https://stemcells.nih.gov/ (site accessed 23/11/2020).

Public Health England (2018) Commissioning local HIV, sexual and reproductive health services. Available from: www.gov.uk/guidance/commissioning-regional-and-local-sexual-health-services#contents (site accessed 21/11/2020).

3   Losses in reproductive years

Infertility

For many couples, an inability to have a baby can represent the loss of hopes and dreams for the future. Consequently, the intimacy of sex is potentially fraught with challenge, often becoming performance to order, rather than driven by sexual desire. Men and women under this sort of pressure can find it hard to voice their feelings about what sex has become. The fear of adding further upset to an already complex and delicate situation perpetuates the silence. Frustration and anger can manifest as sexual dysfunction, such as loss of sexual desire, erectile dysfunction or an inability to orgasm, which may have serious implications for the relationship.

> **MIKE: A CARRIAGE OF INJUSTICE**
>
> Mike was a successful 37-year-old businessman who requested psychosexual therapy for erectile difficulties. At the outset, Mike conveyed his admiration and respect for his wife, but seemed reluctant to talk about the relationship. The difficulties with his erections had worsened over time and this made him feel very low. When asked by the therapist how his wife reacted to the loss of erections, he whispered, 'She gets furious with me, passes bitter comments and then she won't speak to me for days!'
>
> When the counsellor asked how Mike felt about this, he said that he forgave her because she was so desperate to have a baby and they had been trying for such a long time. The therapist asked again how he felt about being talked to in the way he described.
>
> Eventually, Mike allowed himself to let go of his confused feelings of self-blame, shame and guilt over his inability to perform. In the safe space of the consultation, hesitantly, he was able to express

> his anger towards his wife at what appeared to be her disregard of his feelings during this pressured time. As he developed the courage to share his difficult feelings more directly with his wife, a renewed kindness and understanding developed and his ability to sustain his erections once again surprised and delighted them both.

REFLECT

In this instance, Mike's anger was blocking his sexual function, but with support and his own developing insight, he was able to share his reality with his wife.

RESPOND

There are so many areas of life in which we expect that things will get worse for us or we will cause harm to someone else if we speak out. At every level, as HPs, it is helpful if we can give permission to the people we are helping, to our colleagues and within other relationships to share what may be difficult to say.

Miscarriage

As with so many losses, although common, miscarriage of a pregnancy is an act of nature beyond personal control. The loss of a baby before 24 weeks' gestation is known as miscarriage. It can represent a profound loss for those involved, and this grief needs to be recognised and valued.

> ### SERENA'S SADNESS
>
> Serena, in her late thirties, was referred for psychosexual therapy by her GP due to a lack of sexual desire. She had been married for ten years and clearly loved her husband but he was devastated that she didn't want sex. They had been trying for a baby for six years and had experienced three failed attempts at in-vitro fertilisation (IVF). Previously, sex had been enjoyable, but for the last few months she simply couldn't face it.

When the therapist asked how Serena felt about her inability to conceive, she sobbed great tears and said her life and mood were governed by her menstrual cycle: after her period had finished, she was filled with the hope that this time she would fall pregnant. She and her husband would have sex at the optimal time for conception, but a few weeks later when her next period started she would feel an overwhelming sense of grief for the hoped-for child. The therapist suggested that she sounded exhausted by this recurring cycle and asked what Serena felt when she had sex. Serena began to cry again and with the help of the therapist recognised the enormity of her sadness.

REFLECT

Many people, like Serena, find themselves dealing with the effects of underlying loss in its various guises and only slowly start to appreciate how unaddressed grief can affect sexual enjoyment and physical function.

RESPOND

In our experience family, friends and HPs may offer support through reassurance, but does reassurance alone allow or help a person to grieve? Allowing an expression of emotion in the brief moment could reduce the need for antidepressant or anxiety medications in the future.

EMILY: WHEN REASSURANCE BECOMES PAINFUL

Seventeen-year-old Emily attended a sexual health clinic as she had been experiencing painful sex. As her results were all negative, the sexual health advisor (SHA) asked Emily when sex had first become painful. Emily thought it had started about six months previously, but was not sure why. When asked if anything significant had happened around that time, Emily recalled that she had miscarried an unplanned pregnancy. She added that her GP had been kind, reassuring her that miscarriages were common and telling her she had plenty of time to have a baby in the future.

> The SHA wondered if, in this reassurance, Emily's true feelings about the miscarriage had not been explored. She asked Emily to describe what had happened to her, but Emily avoided the question by saying, 'You don't want to know about it. It was horrible!' Sensing the importance of this to Emily, the SHA responded, 'I *do* want to know.' Emily described the pain and the horror of seeing large blood clots coming out of her. She was scared and alone but too frightened to call for help. The SHA and Emily then spent some time discussing the initial shock of the pregnancy, followed soon after by its loss.
>
> A follow-up appointment was arranged to address the painful sex, but Emily cancelled it on the day, leaving a message saying her sex life was now 'all good'.

REFLECT

The reassurance Emily had received from her GP, although well meaning, proved to be detrimental as it blocked the recognition and expression of her grief, making it harder for her to bear. We have discovered that any unexpressed loss can manifest as physical symptoms. For Emily, it was painful sex that followed the unexpected trauma.

RESPOND

In a one-to-one engagement, we have found that allowing patients the space to express the previously unspeakable can quickly become a vehicle for change. Acknowledging the very real impact of trauma on the body and subsequent emotional reactions can form part of the physical and emotional healing process.

Disruption of childbirth

Pregnancy and childbirth are naturally significant life events for parents, relatives and friends. All will have spent some time anticipating the new arrival. The experience of physical and emotional changes during pregnancy and childbirth may leave the individual subject to many conflicting emotions, particularly if the pregnancy was not planned, which at times can be confusing. In our experience, exposure to the excitement, anticipated pain and uncertainty of labour can have a lasting impact on an individual's sexual confidence and/or a couple's intimacy.

> **RAJ AND JEN: NOT SEEN BUT HEARD**
>
> A health visitor (HV) went to the home of Raj and Jen, who had recently had their first baby. At the previous visit Jen had mentioned that Raj had been a bit withdrawn since the birth. When Jen left the room the HV took the opportunity to ask Raj how he felt about the delivery. He replied he had been delighted with the birth of a son. However, he then hesitated for a moment and the HV noticed he had turned quite pale. Almost in a whisper he said, 'I felt physically sick. I can still hear the crunch, crunch of the scissors cutting her to let the baby out. I've been too frightened to get close to her since!' When the HV voiced that such an experience must have been difficult, Raj's colour returned. He looked up and said, 'I feel so relieved telling you. I couldn't tell Jen. I just didn't want to upset her with my stupid feelings.'
>
> With the accepting support of the HV, Raj was able to discuss his 'stupid feelings', which over time helped him to relax and get close to his partner again.

REFLECT

Some subjects may be difficult to discuss even if a childbirth has been a happy event. We have learned that unspoken feelings can create distance and misunderstandings which can affect intimacy and sexual expression.

RESPOND

In our experience, taking a moment during a routine consultation to reflect on the childbirth experience, as with Raj and Jen, may prevent an interim sexual difficulty from becoming a long-term problem.

> **UNREACHABLE ROSIE**
>
> A midwife was looking after Rosie, a first-time mother, and her partner during labour. In order to assess the progress of the labour and guard against an umbilical cord prolapse, she needed to perform a vaginal examination. (An umbilical cord prolapse involves

the cord emerging from the uterus either with or before the presenting part of the baby, which can compromise blood flow to the baby. It occurs in about 1 per cent of births.) However, this proved an impossible task as Rosie clamped her legs tightly together and retreated anxiously up the bed. The midwife felt very uncomfortable and believed that, if she were to continue, it would feel like an assault on Rosie. Rosie eventually consented to an epidural injection with anaesthetic to numb the pain (sometimes known as spinal block), but she was still unable to relax enough to allow a vaginal examination. At this point the midwife wondered how Rosie had managed to become pregnant and put the question to the couple. Her husband replied wearily, 'I honestly don't know. We've been together ten years and we've never been able to do it properly.'

The midwife discussed this challenging situation with the team. As the labour could not be assessed adequately, they decided they had no option but to perform a Caesarean section. This unexpected, unprecedented experience so troubled the midwife that she visited the couple on the postnatal ward the next day and urged them to seek help for their sexual difficulty as soon as they felt able.

REFLECT

This case had such a profound effect on the midwife that she sought out psychosexual training to enable her to respond more effectively in the future and undertook psychosexual skills development with the Association of Psychosexual Nursing (Cort, 2003).

RESPOND

Further training for healthcare professionals in the UK can be accessed through the Institute of Psychosexual Medicine (IPM), the College of Sex and Relationship Therapy (COSRT) and other validated providers.

Near-death experiences and stillbirth

The physical and emotional trauma of delivering a stillborn baby or a baby that dies during childbirth is barely imaginable. Such a loss can affect all family members, friends and acquaintances as well as those who have provided obstetric care (see Jamie's case study, below).

Stillbirth is the term for infant death after 24 full weeks of foetal development. Latest figures suggest that this occurs in approximately 0.5 per cent of all pregnancies in England (NHS, n.d.). Fortunately, midwives are highly trained to spot any warning signs during pregnancy and delivery, and they offer invaluable support and guidance regarding what can be done to minimise the risk. Without this care, rates of stillbirth would be far higher.

We have learned that the fear of not knowing what to say or how to respond can freeze relationships. In addition, being close to someone else's grief can rekindle uninvited memories of personal loss and revive feelings of anger and blame. Similarly, in our experience, a 'near death' during labour or delivery that results in a loss of personal control can profoundly affect relationships and sexual intimacy. Jamie's and Nuala's stories illustrate this.

JAMIE'S TERROR

Jamie, a young woman of 28, was accessing antenatal care in the early stages of her third pregnancy. The midwife immediately realised that she needed to pay close attention as Jamie appeared agitated and irritable, avoiding eye contact. During the history taking, it transpired that Jamie had undergone a termination of pregnancy at the age of 17 and a stillbirth due to genetic abnormality at the age of 25, so it was hardly surprising that this pregnancy was causing her considerable anxiety. The midwife gently requested more information about Jamie's previous experiences and asked if they might be affecting her attitude towards carrying another baby. Jamie immediately started to sob, tears dropping into her lap. The midwife sat quietly until Jamie looked up with a start, her fists clenched and her eyes flashing with anger. She revealed that she had agreed to the abortion at 17 because her step-mother had convinced her she would be unable to cope with raising a baby. Thereafter, she had felt restless and couldn't settle in any job. She had also had frequent unprotected sex without any pleasure before finally finding a loving partner in her early twenties and trying to start a family. However, at this point in her story, Jamie's rage started to bubble up again and she almost shouted, 'But I couldn't manage to keep that one either! I'm no good, I'm no good. What's the point? How will I ever keep this baby?' The midwife allowed Jamie's rage and tears to continue until they subsided.

With Jamie's permission, the midwife arranged early support from the community midwife and suggested that both Jamie and her partner should attend her next appointment with the obstetric consultant as this would give them an opportunity to discuss any concerns. Following this simple intervention and further signposting, Jamie began to sleep better.

REFLECT

Jamie was so full of distress that her demeanour could have been interpreted as 'difficult'. If this had not been addressed, it may well have generated negative feelings among those who were trying to support her through the pregnancy.

RESPOND

A few moments have the potential to change the course of a major life event. Devoting just a little time to learn what is really going on, even during busy clinics, can pay great dividends.

Near-death experiences of any kind can lead to unresolved negative emotions that can impact on relationships if they remain unspoken. Therefore, the ongoing stress and automatic, self-protecting physical and emotional responses must be acknowledged and understood to allow a person to live again in the moment with greater freedom (see Figure 1.1 in Chapter 1).

NUALA'S MOURNING

Following increasingly frequent arguments with her partner, Nuala, in her late twenties and the mother of two small children aged three years and 18 months, asked her GP for help regarding her loss of sexual desire. After a preliminary medical screen which showed no hormonal abnormality, she was referred to a psychosexual therapist.

Nuala felt that her relationship was good aside from the lack of sex, which was the cause of the arguments. She was unclear as to when she had started to avoid sex and why, but assumed that it must have been due to physical exhaustion. After all, she was looking after two toddlers full time.

The counsellor asked Nuala when she had last had intercourse. She admitted that she felt numb and unresponsive, so she and her partner had attempted sex only a couple of times since the birth of their second child. The therapist immediately asked about the last pregnancy and delivery, and Nuala responded that she had enjoyed the pregnancy enormously and she and her partner were both thrilled to have a girl. The counsellor sensed that she was avoiding any discussion of the delivery and put the question to her again. With a sigh, Nuala quietly recalled a moment when she had feared for her own and her baby's life. Then she began to cry uncontrollably.

After a few moments, the therapist acknowledged Nuala's distress and asked if she had ever talked this through with her partner. She replied that they had never spoken of it. At the following session Nuala reported that the couple had talked long into the night and shared for the first time the terrifying memory of that moment during the delivery. Having spoken in such an intimate way, Nuala found herself sexually aroused and surprised by the return of sexual feelings towards her partner.

REFLECT

Sexual feeling can be disturbed by traumatic experiences, such as miscarriage, termination, stillbirth and complex childbirth. In addition, memories of sexual assault, sexual abuse, domestic violence, emotional abuse or delivery of a child with complex needs can resurface during the antenatal or postnatal period.

RESPOND

It is important to listen and to identify the most likely source of the distress. In addition, the HP should have some knowledge of local specialist therapy or counselling services that may be offered to the patient at some point in the future, including their waiting times and referral procedures.

References

Cort, E. (2003). Psychosexual awareness: an invaluable skill for nurses. *Nursing in Practice*, 11, pp. 74–76.

NHS (n.d.) Stillbirth. Available from: www.nhs.uk/conditions/stillbirth/ (site accessed 21/11/2020).

Further reading

Royal College of Obstetricians and Gynaecologists (2015) Umbilical cord prolapse in late pregnancy. Available from: www.rcog.org.uk/globalassets/documents/patients/patient-information-leaflets/pregnancy/pi-umbilical-cord-prolapse-in-late-pregnancy.pdf (site accessed 23/11/2020).

4 Unexpected outcomes and sexual development

Physical difference

The impact on parents following the news and birth of a physically disabled baby can be unexpected. Unspoken feelings of guilt and shame can remain between the couple, affecting their relationship. As well as their own shock, they may have to manage other people's reactions of disappointment and pity. In the longer term, we have seen evidence of sexual problems directly related to the fear of having another family member affected by a similar genetic disorder contributing to delayed ejaculation, failure of erection or loss of sexual desire. However, the opposite can also occur, whereby the challenge of the situation can bring couples closer together in the care and love of their precious child.

> ### JULIE AND SAM'S PROTECTED LOVE
>
> Julie had wanted to be a mother of many children from her earliest memory, and after she married Sam the couple soon conceived. Their families and friends were delighted. However, at the 20-week scan a growth abnormality was noted and a more invasive test was suggested to confirm it. Julie and Sam knew the risks of this test and wanted to keep their baby, so they declined the procedure. Thereafter, though, between them and individually, there was much soul searching, low feelings and sadness.
>
> Once relatives and friends heard the news, Julie and Sam also had to cope with their pity, outrage and refusal to believe that the first measures of the baby's development were accurate. Julie and Sam were exhausted and wanted to be left alone.
>
> It was eight months before everyone had adjusted to the fact that Julie and Sam's baby may have physical challenges. At the birth,

> there was quiet acceptance and joy at meeting their first son. The couple, totally wrapped up in his care, found a fierce and protective love which carried them through the following years, especially as their own sexual intimacy could not be their priority.

REFLECT

Recognising the enormity of coping with the birth and ongoing development of a 'less than perfect' baby can represent a significant loss at the outset but can also lead to profound gains over time. At that time sex may not be on the agenda.

RESPOND

We have found it can be helpful for difficult feelings to be heard without presumption or negative judgement. Each person's individual reaction to unexpected circumstances should be respected. Over time, this will strengthen family bonds and support the parents' ability to cope when times are hard. However, it is still important to talk about sex rather than leave it unspoken for too long.

Physical and mental challenges

Fierce protectiveness over a child with a congenital disability is understandable. However, this can be problematic and particularly challenging during adolescence, when the child will develop sexually regardless of their mental age. This can be alarming for parents who are unable to accept their child's emerging sexuality, as it brings a fear of added vulnerability and the potential risk of exploitation.

The emotional sexual development of the young person who has a physical or learning disability from birth may also be blocked by societal attitudes. Equally, it is important for those who provide care to consider that a young person who experiences an acquired disability due to trauma or medical conditions later in life may or may not have had earlier opportunities to be sexually active.

As a child develops, the physical disability may be immediately recognisable or less noticeable, such as a hearing or visual impairment. In either case, others may respond with feelings of discomfort or uncertainty as to how best to communicate with them. Depending on personal experience, people may display a variety of reactions to individuals with physical or communication challenges, such as:

- Speaking louder and slower than necessary
- Using inappropriately simplistic language
- Being overly helpful
- Doing things for the person without asking
- Speaking to a carer rather than the individual

As annoying as these reactions may be, they are usually genuine, if misguided, attempts to help.

MO: SHOUTING TO BE HEARD

Mo was in his early forties and struggling to develop a long-term relationship. Following occasional visits to a commercial sex worker, he regularly attended a sexual health clinic for screening. During one of these visits, he asked the sexual health advisor (SHA) a question. It was a very busy clinic and the SHA became frustrated as Mo's speech was slow and difficult to understand due to his cerebral palsy. Finally, she said, 'Don't worry about it, you will be fine!' and pointed to the door.

Mo leaned forward, took the pen out of her hand and wrote on a piece of paper: 'YOU ARE NOT LISTENING TO ME!'

Full of shame, the SHA shut the door on the busy waiting room and respectfully sat back to listen.

REFLECT

We have found that reflecting on our own prejudices helps us to focus on the individual. Each person has unique needs.

RESPOND

It is important to ask directly how best to communicate before unintentionally causing offence.

> ### LISA'S LOVE LIFE
>
> In her twenties, Lisa sought psychosexual therapy due to her confusion regarding her sexual preferences. On meeting her in the waiting room, the therapist was momentarily overwhelmed by the sight of Lisa's contorted body in a wheelchair. Her first concern was how to manoeuvre Lisa into the consulting room through a busy waiting area and narrow corridor. She also felt mounting apprehension about broaching the subject of sex without knowing Lisa's physical capabilities. And she was anxious about letting Lisa down, especially as she had no previous experience of working with a severely physically disabled patient.
>
> However, Lisa immediately took control of the situation and expertly guided herself and the therapist into the consulting room. As she talked about her thoughts and feelings regarding her sexual concerns, the wheelchair 'disappeared' and the therapeutic relationship began.

REFLECT

In the encounters with Mo and Lisa, despite some disability awareness, one HP was overwhelmed by time pressure that overrode her usual sensitivity, and the other doubted both her patient's and her own ability to manage the situation physically and emotionally. Thankfully, both of the individuals who were seeking help had the courage to take control, and their active collaboration ensured that an effective therapeutic engagement could begin.

RESPOND

It is important not to make assumptions and to understand the personal context before offering any advice.

Acquired physical disability

When a person acquires a physical disability later in life do we assume their sexual feelings disappear and their sex life ceases? Due to the change in circumstances, each person has the potential to re-engage with or develop sexual intimacy if they have the desire to do so. This need should

Unexpected outcomes and sexual development 61

be respected and considered alongside all other needs and challenges. It is also important to be aware of the impact of the acquired changes on their partner and any significant others.

> **STEPH AND TERRY: STEPH'S SECRET**
>
> Steph and Terry were a couple in their early fifties – what should have been the prime of life when they could finally enjoy more leisure time and develop their intimacy. However, Terry then sustained a severe head injury. At first, Steph simply said she was thankful her husband had survived and insisted she had adapted well to his mood swings and the daily physical challenges his condition presented. However, with encouragement from the doctor, she then started to talk about their sex life, which had been intimate and loving prior to the accident. After a while, she became very tearful and sad as she reported that Terry now lacked awareness of other people's feelings, which was particularly upsetting for Steph during intercourse, as it was like having sex with a stranger.
>
> There were many challenges for this couple, but the greatest for Steph was the loss of small acts of intimacy and the familiar connection that she and Terry had shared in the past.

> **MARION'S COVER**
>
> Marion presented as a frail woman and came into the session with a walking frame. She was in her early sixties and told the therapist that she had suffered a stroke 18 months earlier. This had affected the left side of her body, in particular her leg. She talked about how supportive her husband had been and assured the therapist that they still had a strong relationship. However, with sadness, she also reported the loss of their physical relationship, telling the therapist that she just did not feel 'sexy' any more and pointing to the 'useless' left side of her body.
>
> During two follow-up sessions the therapist explored how Marion might allow herself to become a sensual woman again and made suggestions regarding what could help her achieve this. For

instance, as the sight of her disability upset Marion so much, it was suggested that she should consider wearing something that covered her up but still made her feel good.

At the next session Marion reported that she had worn a long negligee, much to her husband's delight, and they had made love. She realised in that moment that their sexual pleasure was about the emotional and physical connection between them, not how her body looked. She cried with relief that she had found this kind of intimacy again.

REFLECT

The examples of Terry and Steph and Marion illustrate how acquired disabilities, seen or unseen, can affect an intimate relationship. Steph and Terry lost their previously shared acts of intimacy and familiar ways, whereas Marion felt shame over the physical changes to her body, which had led to a loss of sexual desire. It is important to remember that the acquired disability may present profound challenges to day-to-day living in itself. But these two cases reveal that it can also jeopardise emotional and sexual closeness, which in turn can have profound implications for the person's ability to cope.

RESPOND

We have found that it is important to consider not only the impact of an acquired disability on daily life but also how it may impact upon relationships that are vital to a person's or a couple's wellbeing.

Learning-disabled challenges

Regardless of mental capacity, physical changes will continue during puberty. Therefore, physical sexual development should not be ignored, even though carers may experience anxiety over the emerging sexuality as well as fears of potential exploitation and harm to the individual. Those who have cared for a young person since childhood often find it difficult to embrace his or her emerging sexual development, as the caring role demands significant adjustment and inevitable change.

Some of the blocks to facilitating healthy sexual development are:

- Concerns over capacity to consent
- Fear that sex education will encourage sexual activity, which may result in a pregnancy or a sexually transmitted infection
- The attitudes or cultural beliefs of care workers who find the concept of sexual activity among learning-disabled people unacceptable
- Fear of raising the sexual expectations of the learning-disabled person
- Fear of encouraging socially unacceptable sexual behaviours
- An assumption that the individual will be unable to understand contraception and safer-sex information

It is essential to balance any risk of harm against maintaining a respectful approach towards the individuality and independence of the learning-disabled person.

REFLECT

In many environments, particularly where health or social care is provided, addressing the sexual needs of individuals can be a challenge not only for parents and family members but also for HPs. Are people with a learning disability, or the appearance of one, given adequate opportunities to talk about their sexual hopes and fears?

RESPOND

Acknowledging frustrations and low mood and asking what is upsetting the learning-challenged person can lead to further discussion, encourage autonomy and enhance the individual's wellbeing. A candid discussion among family members, HPs and the individual may help all concerned to work together to support and embrace the learning-challenged person's sexuality as safely as possible, rather than ignore or disallow it.

A GOOD NIGHT OUT

A group of people with learning disabilities wanted to explore a local night club to dance, have fun and maybe find a partner. Prior to this, two or three had ventured out to experience the local nightclub scene, but they were hurt by the response of other young people and their own unrealistic expectations.

> As a group, they discussed using established dating agencies, but concerned health professionals were worried about their vulnerability and the possibility of sexual exploitation. So, with professional help, they set up a specialist dating agency that paid careful attention to registration and membership. This paved the way to many enjoyable nights out.

REFLECT

This group of young people and their carers worked together as a team. The result was life-enhancing for all concerned.

RESPOND

It may be beneficial for HPs and individuals to find (or establish) a local dating and friendship agency that caters exclusively to the needs of young people and adults with learning difficulties.

Further reading

Lehmann, K. (2005) The provision of sexual health care for adult women with learning disabilities. *Journal of Community Nursing*, 19(9), pp. 10–14.

5 Mental health

Sexual function can be adversely affected among those experiencing mental health conditions, including anxiety and depression. There are many forms of mental illness, ranging from mild to severe. At one end of the spectrum, mental illness can manifest in part as sexual disinhibition. At the other, for example when someone is anxious or depressed, it can lead to a total loss of sexual desire and other issues. Moreover, these problems can be complicated by medication. Whilst antidepressants and other drugs may improve mood and reduce extremes of experience, they can also exacerbate conditions such as erectile dysfunction and further inhibit sexual desire.

Obsessive Compulsive Disorder

Obsessive Compulsive Disorder (OCD) is often characterised by repetitive patterns of behaviour to reduce the anxiety of perceived danger. For example, hand-washing to eliminate microbes or checking that doors are locked against unwelcome invasion may indicate problems with intimate relationships, such as difficulties with sexual arousal, low sex drive, feelings of discontent, fear of sex or disgust when thinking about sexual activities due to fears of contamination. In addition, previous sexual violence or developing fears relating to cultural or religious views on perceived sinful or prohibited sexual behaviour are amongst the challenges we have experienced in psychosexual practice linked to OCD.

> **WAITING FOR SABRINA**
>
> Sabrina, in her early thirties, attended a consultation with a psychosexual therapist. On initial presentation, she was fashionably dressed and seemingly confident. She declared that she loved her partner

of ten years, David, but admitted that she was unable to allow any spontaneous sexual contact with him. This was the reason for her visit, as it was impacting negatively on their relationship.

Sabrina appeared to be a 'successful' and 'in control' young woman, which led the therapist to ask her how things were at home. Sabrina replied that she needed to maintain order and always kept their home spotless. The mention of 'order' alerted the therapist to consider what sex might be like for the couple, so she asked Sabrina to describe their last sexual connection. Sabrina talked of the previous morning: David had leaned over to kiss her on the lips as she was waking up, but she had immediately rushed to the bathroom to clean her teeth and shower. The therapist detected an atmosphere of sterility and isolation in the room while Sabrina was speaking, and suggested that her need to be clean had broken what might have been a warm and intimate moment.

On reflection with Sabrina, the therapist intimated that the current situation was rather sad for the couple. Although this comment upset her, Sabrina replied with recognition and some relief, 'I hate doing that to him, but I have never felt able to tell him why. Maybe I'll be able to tell him now.'

Previously, Sabrina had visited her GP for help with low sexual desire, but during the therapy sessions it became apparent that her avoidance of sex was due to a form of Obsessive Compulsive Disorder. The therapist worked with the couple over five further sessions to manage this and enable them to move forward. As Sabrina became more accepting of herself as less than perfect but more than good enough, spontaneous intimacy improved for the couple.

REFLECT

Sabrina sought help for what she perceived to be low sexual desire, but further exploration revealed that this problem was actually linked to her OCD.

RESPOND

In practice we have found that it is even more important to discover the source of the sexual problem when there are mental health challenges.

Equally, unwanted sexual experiences that remain unspoken can be at the root of mental health distress. Looking at and learning from the whole person can help the therapist and patient to determine the best way forward.

Anxiety and depression

We all experience low moods from time to time, but for most of us the feelings pass in due course. Depression, by contrast, is a perpetual low mood that affects everyday life. A 'normal' life can still be led, but depression makes many things more of a struggle and less satisfying. Sensations of hopelessness, tearfulness, despair, agitation, emptiness and numbness may be experienced. Similarly, anxiety is common when coping with stressful events or major life changes. People living with anxiety often experience restlessness, worry, low concentration, sleeplessness, dizziness and even heart palpitations. Anxiety and depression are often found in combination, but not always.

Each person's reduced mental health will be uniquely experienced. Asking about the personal experience of anxiety or depression can be helpful within a relationship as well as during therapy in order for the appropriate support to be tailored to the individual. In the UK, MIND can provide information on and support for many common mental health challenges (Medical Investigation of Neurodevelopmental Disorders, n.d.).

LEILA: BLINDED TO THE EVIDENCE

Following a recent marital break-up, Leila went to see her GP in a tearful, anxious and low state. The GP appeared uncomfortable at Leila's distress and immediately offered her a prescription for antidepressants, which he advised would make her feel calmer. As Leila left, the GP reassured her that if she felt better with the tablets, she could request a repeat prescription without needing to see him again. Leila chose not take the tablets because she didn't feel this was the solution to her suffering.

REFLECT

This type of distress may be anticipated in the light of a significant life event.

RESPOND

We may consider what emotions might be expected as a natural physical response to unexpected life events but we should never make assumptions. Validating difficult feelings may support the individual to cope before the offer of a prescription is required.

> ### ZENAB: WHAT GOOD IS A WEEKEND AWAY?
>
> Zenab, a busy working mother, visited her doctor's surgery complaining of loss of sexual desire, low mood, tearfulness and feelings of hopelessness. The GP advised that all she really needed was a break in the form of a good weekend away. Zenab left feeling more hopeless as she could not afford the time away nor understand how this would help in the long term.

REFLECT

On this occasion the GP did not rush to prescribe medication, but did she really listen to Zenab or rather make an assumption based on personal experience?

RESPOND

Briefly exploring feelings of hopelessness can provide the necessary evidence or insight to proceed with a more appropriate patient-focused intervention.

The cases of Leila and Zenab illustrate how similar presentations may need different approaches. Leila may have benefited from having her shock and distress simply acknowledged, whereas the opposite was true for Zenab, who may well have benefited from some form of medication and counselling. Unfortunately, neither woman received an effective intervention, in part because neither was asked what she felt she needed. No choice was given in the management of their symptoms, leaving them both feeling shut down and no nearer to a resolution.

It is easier to learn from case studies such as these on reflection after the event, and our reflectionsare in no way meant as criticisms of professional colleagues. Such challenging exposure from our own and others' learnings regarding personal encounters with individuals can, if we can bear it, enhance professional sensitivity, ultimately improving patient outcomes.

REFLECT

Research, confirmed by our own experience, suggests that the pressures of primary care may lead GPs to become over-reliant on medication to alleviate moderate mental health disorders before identifying the potential cause with the individual. The pressure to prescribe may also be fuelled by the patient's expectation of leaving the surgery with medication. Research into patient experience develops an appreciation of these pressures and assumptions during medical consultations and the value of hearing the patient's perspective and the outcomes they seek from those consultations (Dwamena et al., 2009).

RESPOND

Regarding the expected human response to life events such as sadness, pain, anxiety and anger, recovery over time with empathic support and follow-up takes its natural course. In addition, a talking therapy may be helpful for the individual who feels 'stuck'. If such emotions are not acknowledged sensitively, and if they are inhibited by medication, we have seen long-term physical effects within sexual relationships. Nevertheless, in situations where there is unresolved grief, it is sometimes helpful to use medication and a talking therapy in combination to achieve a better outcome. It is always helpful to find out about counselling providers in the local area to offer patient choice, should the need arise.

At times, individuals have different communication needs, moods and styles which the HP should endeavour to recognise as soon as possible. Aspects of Autistic Spectrum Disorder are discussed below to illustrate communication differences.

Autistic traits

An Autistic Spectrum Disorder (ASD) can cause problems with communication and social interaction, restricted interests, repetitive patterns of behaviour and difficulties with creating and maintaining relationships (see National Autistic Society, n.d.). In many cases of those who come forward for specialist help, we find that the challenge of a sexual relationship can exacerbate rather than mitigate autistic traits.

CLIVE'S MISCONNECTION

A 50-year-old man, Clive, entered the therapy room in shorts on a cold January day. He disclosed that he was in his early thirties before he lost his virginity, with his current partner. During the first couple of sessions Clive admitted that he didn't really enjoy 'it' because he thought 'it' was dirty. He didn't even like the feel of his partner's skin under his hands. The therapist suggested they should invite his partner to the next session. She agreed to attend and described feeling unconnected during sex. She said that Clive patted her in an almost childlike way, and it was obvious that he was not enjoying the sexual activity either. This was clearly a difficult situation for the couple and the therapist could see how upsetting it was for each of them.

Over the course of subsequent sessions the therapist began to realise that Clive was displaying some ASD traits. Basic tasks such as trying to allocate quality time for each other were difficult because of Clive's set routines, which he needed to follow each evening. Eventually, the therapist reached the conclusion that the couple's sexual differences were too great to resolve and she was driven to ask what kept them together. The couple joined forces in their reply: the bond between them was more important than their sexual relationship; they loved each other and wanted to stay together even if they could not find a solution to their sexual problems.

During the final session the therapist asked Clive, 'Why do you wear shorts when it's so cold?'

Clive replied, 'I hate the feel of anything on my legs. As soon as I get home from work I take my trousers off and put on a skirt.'

REFLECT

Clive's final comment made perfect sense to both the therapist and his partner as it highlighted his aversion to any type of touch and consequently why he found it so difficult to enjoy sex. Of course, in addition, the therapist might have interpreted it as an admission of transvestism, but on further sensitive enquiry she concluded that this was not the case.

LOVELY LEONARD

Leonard was a quiet, shy man in his late twenties. He wore clothes that were older than his years and he was extremely polite and courteous. He disclosed that he had never had a relationship and that he was still a virgin. He had developed Obsessive Compulsive Disorder related to a deep-seated fear of upsetting 'God'. He had read the Bible and researched Christianity when he was about 12 years old and had become obsessive and anxious about adhering to the Ten Commandments. This had led to outspoken questioning of his peers at school, with the consequence that he was shunned and ignored. At this point, the therapist started to wonder whether Leonard had some autistic traits. These became more apparent when he talked about his father's behaviour. Eventually, his anxiety had worsened and he had spent a lot of time at home with his parents and less time in school.

Leonard explained that both parents had recently died, and he now lived in the parental home with his older brother. He said he really wanted a girlfriend, but his obsession with religion had meant he had not experienced any teenage relationships as he could not consider sex outside of marriage. He also disclosed that he had masturbated on a regular basis since the age of 12. He did this in the shower or bath while wearing his clothes because he enjoyed the sensation of the wet fabric against his genitals. This provided him with some comfort but it was also a source of guilt and shame.

During the consultations, the therapist noted Leonard's fragility and naivety, and she often felt as if she were talking to a young boy. When he discussed his parents' deaths, it was clear that he had blocked all emotion. However, during one session, he was very upset as his rabbit had just died. He was shocked at how distressed he felt and the therapist reflected with him that perhaps the loss of his pet had unblocked his grief over the loss of his parents.

The therapy focused on moving Leonard forward. He joined a Christian dating agency and asked the therapist if they could write a dating profile together. He eventually met a young woman and the therapist told him she was delighted for him. He arrived for his final session in jeans and with highlights in his hair, at last appearing his true age. The therapist felt her chest bursting with pride.

REFLECT

It is important to acknowledge and record our feelings and emotional responses to the people we see. These can be both positive and negative, so clinical case supervision is vital to explore whether we ourselves are blocking the therapeutic space. (See Chapter 13.)

RESPOND

Again, it is crucial to remain open to the personal perspective of the individual during a consultation as this can provide a valuable indicator as to the most appropriate way forward. We can see autistic traits in both Clive and Leonard – one detested touch of any kind whilst the other secretly embraced sensation.

References

Dwamena, F.C., Lyles, J.S., Frankel, R.M. and Smith, R.C. (2009) In their own words: qualitative study of high-utilising primary care patients with medically unexplained symptoms. *BMC Family Practitioner*, 10. Available from: https://bmcfampract.biomedcentral.com/articles/10.1186/1471-2296-10-67 (site accessed 01/02/2021).

Medical Investigation of Neurodevelopmental Disorders (n.d.) Types of mental health problems. Available from: www.mind.org.uk/information-support/types-of-mental-health-problems/ (site accessed 23/11/2020).

National Autistic Society (n.d.) What is autism? Available from: www.autism.org.uk/advice-and-guidance/what-is-autism (site accessed 21/11/2020).

NHS (n.d.) Obsessive Compulsive Disorder (OCD.) Available from: www.nhs.uk/conditions/obsessive-compulsive-disorder-ocd/symptoms/ (site accessed 21/11/2020).

Further reading

NHS (n.d.) Mental health and wellbeing. Available from: www.nhs.uk/conditions/stress-anxiety-depression/ (site accessed 23/11/2020).

NHS England (n.d.) Adult improving access to psychological therapies programme. Available from: www.england.nhs.uk/mental-health/adults/iapt/ (site accessed 01/02/2021).

Psych Central (n.d.) Autism. Available from: https://psychcentral.com/autism/ (site accessed 23/11/2020).

6 Gender identity, sexuality and difference in sexual desire

Increasing numbers of individuals who are confused about their gender identity, sexuality and differences in sexual desire are seeking support and help. Some people can find it hard, if not impossible, to meet society's gender expectations, leading to isolation and unhappiness. This concern is by no means a new phenomenon and in some societies, over time, the boundaries between the common conceptions of male and female behaviours have been broadened to accommodate and accept difference. When a person cannot or refuses to fit the expected norm of a male or female role in society, they can feel that there is something unacceptable to others or even to themselves. For further clarity, Paz Galupo, Stuart and Siegal (2015: p. 549) outline the inclusivity of the generally accepted term 'transgender':

> Although the experiences of transgender, transsexual, and gender variant individuals may be distinct, they are often considered under a common umbrella term of *transgender* or *trans**. Individuals who fall under the trans umbrella may include cross-dressers, transvestites, transsexuals, drag kings and queens, as well as individuals who identify as transwomen, transmen, bigender, two-spirit, androgynous, genderqueer, gender nonconforming, and gender variant.

Many pronouns are used to indicate a transgender or gender variant identity, with the most common being 'they', 'their' and 'them'. During consultations it is important to agree upon the preferred pronoun with each individual.

JACKIE AND ICHIKA: CROSS-PURPOSES

Jack, a 33-year-old transgender male, presented for psychosexual therapy. Previously known as Jackie, as a teenager Jack had felt he was in the wrong body, which had resulted in low moods and isolation. However, at the time, he was told he would have to wait until he was older before he could begin gender identity treatment. In the interim, he busied himself with a career, met Ichika and fell in love. He felt he was honest about his intention to physically transition from female to male from the outset of their relationship. After a few months, they moved in together and the reassignment process began, starting with gender dysphoria counselling, which Ichika occasionally attended. By now, Jack was binding his chest to appear more masculine, and he went on to have a bilateral mastectomy.

Shortly after Jack's operation, Ichika was diagnosed with breast cancer, which necessitated a single mastectomy of her own. Thereafter, their relationship started to falter. Jack began hormone therapy and enjoyed the process of becoming more masculine by the day, but he and Ichika were drifting apart and eventually separated.

The counsellor spent some time exploring the relationship breakup. Jack was finding it extremely difficult, but he had no doubt in his mind that he was moving towards being in the 'right' body. He finally realised the sexual impact this must have had on Ichika, who had never been attracted to men and could not tolerate being in a relationship with one. Jack had also been unaware of how his changed gender identity had deeply affected her in relation to her health. Serious illness had forced Ichika to accept the removal of one of her breasts, whereas Jack had actively requested a mastectomy and been delighted by the outcome. His joy had merely compounded Ichika's grief over what she viewed as the devastating loss of an important aspect of her femininity. The couple had not recognised this hidden distress and their differences could not be resolved. The end of the relationship was the sad but inevitable outcome.

REFLECT

Despite Ichika's awareness of the planned gender reassignment from the outset of her relationship with Jack, the reality of the process impacted irreversibly on their intimacy. After they had breast surgery for two very different reasons, Ichika found it unacceptable that Jack celebrated his choice even though he knew that she had been left with no choice – she needed the surgery to save her life. That said, Jack may have argued precisely the same thing.

RESPOND

Whilst an individual may consider gender reassignment to be the only way forward for them, the impact can profoundly affect a long-term sexual relationship. The partner will need to transition in other ways to accommodate the change, which can be a complicated and challenging process for some. For example, following Jack's transition, he and Ichika were no longer a lesbian couple. A couple and their families may need support to work through the consequences of a proposed gender change and its social impact. See the next two case studies for further discussion of the complexities that may arise within families as well as the internal struggles that some individuals face.

RICHARD'S RESPONSIBILITY

Richard, in his late fifties and suffering with low mood and anxiety, was referred to the local Wellbeing Service following a suicide attempt. He was referred for psychosexual counselling immediately after assessment to address the long-term gender identity issues that seemed to be at the heart of his desperation.

Richard was at his wits' end after coming out to his wife as trans female, which she had found totally unacceptable. There had been no further discussion other than he was to tell no one, especially not their children. Richard felt that he could no longer pretend to be someone he was not, and this emotional turmoil led to his attempt to take his own life.

The therapist continued to gain insights into Richard's private thoughts and unhappiness about his outwardly male gender identity in the context of his early life relationship experiences. Furthermore, she heard that he had experienced little sexual desire for his wife over the years and lived in fear of her angry outbursts when she did not get her own way. The couple eventually agreed to a trial separation within the home, and although Richard was heartbroken, he adhered to his wife's instruction not to tell their children about his trans female identity and feelings.

The therapist continued to explore Richard's thoughts about keeping the reality from his children and the potentially harmful consequences for their parent–child relationships. He was in an almost impossible position as he had to deal with the very real of possibility of being thrown out of the marital home, with nowhere to go, if he told them. The therapist reminded him of the emotional harm his continued silence might do to his children should they find out about his trans status from someone else, and encouraged him to take responsibility as a parent as well as for himself.

ANDROGYNOUS AMY

Amy was referred by her GP for psychosexual counselling in the hope that this might alleviate her gender confusion, low mood and anxiety. Soon to leave home for university, she arrived for her first session dressed in black clothing that made her appear androgynous; she seemed agile but at the same time anxious and fragile. The therapist immediately felt that she should proceed gently with her.

Amy admitted that she struggled to 'fit in' with any group at school and had no close friends. This left her feeling dismayed as she increasingly isolated herself from her family, with little appetite for anything. Her father, in particular, was worried about her frequent low moods and irritability, but she could not find the words to explain what was worrying her. She told the therapist that she felt terrified about moving away from home.

On further gentle exploration of her inability to fit in, Amy described her confusion: she hated the 'girly' gender identity that all her peers at school seemed to share. Everyone else seemed preoccupied with having sex and finding boyfriends, whereas Amy had no interest in either. They were just not on her radar. She became more desperate to find an answer as to why she felt so different. Nothing made any sense to her, so she had reached the conclusion that something must be seriously wrong with her and she would always be strange.

Over time, it became clear not only that Amy had no interest in sex but also that she was confused by her inability to fit in.

> The therapist discussed Amy's confusion about her gender identity, which she considered non-binary – between male and female – as well as asexual.
>
> At the first session following her first term away at university, Amy reported that she had started to notice some people who seemed similar to her, but she was still keeping very much to herself. She was offered links to non-binary and asexuality internet resources in the hope that these might resonate with her own situation.

REFLECT

Once Amy's low mood and irritability were explored, she was willing to discuss her despair. As Richard's case highlights, there are often complex hurdles to overcome for the individual and those around them.

RESPOND

Theory-based knowledge should never overwhelm our focused listening to what the person is saying about their own reality. The value of therapy, although often unarticulated, is that it can build an essential bridge to the future. A mutually agreed way forward is more likely to build confidence.

> **FINDING FELICITY**
>
> Eighteen-year-old Felicity was referred for psychosexual therapy to address her gender confusion. She arrived for her first session looking very feminine in skinny jeans, T-shirt and woolly hat.
>
> Felicity advised the therapist that she wanted to be seen as non-binary (also previously known as 'genderqueer') – that is, neither male nor female – to be considered gender fluid and not to be termed 'she' or 'he' but 'they'. The therapist discovered that Felicity was a much-wanted only daughter as her mother had experienced several miscarriages before she was born. She was also the only grandchild in the family.

> Felicity talked about how they wanted to be male. They hated their breasts and had bound them to render them less noticeable. They also got angry when people were confused and did not know if they were a boy or a girl. However, by hiding their breasts and dressing in non-gender-specific clothes, whilst keeping the name Felicity, others were left not knowing how to react and felt a need to ask. Felicity had not had a full sexual experience, but they acknowledged that they were attracted to boys.
>
> The therapist explored whether there was a high expectation of Felicity to be the perfect daughter and granddaughter, and wondered if that had led to a kind of rebellion which now caused the family and Felicity great distress. The therapy continued by exploring Felicity's anger around gender identity and discomfort over her place in the family and looked for ways to manage social expectations that would be less hurtful to their sense of wellbeing.

REFLECT

Developing a sense of self that enhances a young person's wellbeing is a natural and essential process in human development. However, it takes time and is often achieved through trial and error.

Felicity was still exploring their identity and their ambivalence about being female caused confusion to themself and others. By contrast, when Jackie became Jack, he was quite sure about the transition to a male gender identity.

RESPOND

Felicity and Jack are just two examples of the complex journeys that many people have to take towards adjusting to gender identity and sexuality preference. We strongly advocate giving time to the individual and close relatives to explore their own responses and feel any loss as an integral and valid part of the gender change pathway.

Sexual desire and differences in sexual expression

Ever since the 1950s, sexology researchers such as Masters and Johnson have assumed that desire invariably precedes arousal. For women in particular, this has led to feelings of failure if spontaneous sexual desire is not part of their personal experience. More recently, it has been shown that cultural context and the quality of relationships are more important factors for women, followed by physical closeness. Thereafter, sexual arousal and a subsequent desire for sexual connection tend to develop naturally (Nagoski, 2015; Gurney, 2020). We argue that this is equally applicable to men who fail to experience spontaneous sexual desire at certain times in their lives and in certain contexts.

Differences in level of desire, sexual preference and past experiences all contribute to personal identity, which can change and develop over time.

ANDERS' REBELLION

Anders was a 28-year-old gay man who attended for psychosexual therapy as he was concerned that he may not actually be gay. He had told his parents that his preference was for other men at the age of 16, and they had been extremely supportive and allowed him to bring his boyfriends home without question. However, Anders was confused because he had developed feelings for a close female friend; indeed, he thought he might be falling in love with her. During the therapy he reflected that perhaps his attraction to the same sex was an act of rebellion because he had expected a battle with his parents prior to coming out to them. The fact that they had been so understanding had left him feeling confused.

Anders discussed his concerns at length and in the third session reported that he had spent the night with his female friend. But they had slept next to each other without any sexual contact at all. He learned from this experience that he did not feel any physical attraction towards her, although he really liked her as a person and wanted to be close to her.

The therapist explored the different types of love individuals can feel in certain relationships: for parents, siblings, friends and a sexual partner. After this, Anders felt he did not need further sessions and on leaving informed the therapist with a cheeky grin that he had seen an attractive waiter in a restaurant and they had exchanged numbers.

MARCO'S MANIA

Marco had always felt different from his peers, but he was 53 before he finally started therapy to explore his sexual identity and reduced desire. The therapist understood from him that he was no longer interested in sex with anyone without the use of 'chem sex drugs' (chemical substances that may be used over a long period of time to enhance same-sex sexual drive). He had never had any sexual interest in women.

Through the therapeutic exploration, Marco reluctantly revealed that a man in authority who gave him much-needed support and status as a young child had expressed his affection for him through sexual acts.

In his teenage years, Marco's curiosity about same-sex acts led him to seek out men having sex with other men in the hope of stumbling across a relationship that would fulfil his need for connection. Nevertheless, he never revealed any personal details, always remained anonymous and ensured he never had sex with the same person more than once due to fears that his personal reputation might be shattered. He began dealing in chem sex drugs in order to boost his need to be needed, unable to recognise the resulting self-harm and harm to others that his behaviour represented.

Over time in therapy, Marco recognised his character difference and choice of distance from others as self-protecting against his own vulnerability. More than this, though, as he started to accept his simple longing for community he was able to become a good friend to others. His admission that he had no sexual desire without drugs brought him considerable relief.

REFLECT

The need to develop a personal identity and the links to satisfying arousal and desire are universal. For Anders, the journey was one of rebellion and discovery. By contrast, Marco's voyage was substantially disrupted by an early sexualised relationship with someone who held a position of trust in the community. He eventually found himself engaging in illegal activity and putting others at serious risk by following his own falsely given hopes for connection and recognition. His desire to be close to others having sex rather any desire to connect sexually with another person was an essential part of his story. Therapy allowed Anders to grant himself the freedom he needed to pursue same-sex relationships, and it enabled Marco to acknowledge and accept his own asexuality.

RESPOND

We have found through experience that allowing individuals to tell their own stories and hear them empathically reflected back can generate personal revelation and insight and give them the freedom to make choices for the future that are more congruent with their life values.

TONY/IRENE'S TURMOIL

Tony had been cross-dressing for years with the consent of his wife, Pat, not least because it enhanced his sexual arousal and satisfaction during their love-making. The couple also attended social events with other cross-dressers and their partners. They tended to enjoy these outings as they met people beyond their usual social circle. Tony wondered whether a physical gender identity transition might give him more peace of mind, but in effect he answered his own question because he could not countenance revealing his secret to friends he had known for many years. In addition, he had recently experienced a loss of sexual desire and he missed the intimacy he had previously enjoyed with Pat.

The therapist asked whether Tony had a favourite trans female name. He replied that he liked the name Irene and asked the therapist to use the pronoun 'she' during their sessions. Nevertheless, outwardly, Irene's dress and manner continued to be aligned with the male sex.

Following a discussion about a recent demotion at work and her impending retirement, Irene revealed that the thought of spending more time with Pat had left her feeling as if she wanted to run away.

REFLECT

On further exploration, Irene and the therapist established that the prospect of enforced close contact with Pat's constant health anxiety had triggered Irene's loss of sexual desire.

RESPOND

It is important to follow through with lines enquiry in order to understand the underlying cause of any sexual concern as this leads to recognition and ownership.

Differences in sexual desire and arousal

Many people find it difficult to distinguish between sexual desire and arousal. In a study of individual views on the subject, participants most often felt 'that desire preceded arousal; some felt that desire was "mind" and arousal "body"; and many felt that both desire and arousal were responsive and motivational' (Mitchell, Wellings and Graham, 2014: p. 17). Through our work, we have found that sexual desire and arousal can be enhanced or reduced depending on numerous factors, including physical conditions, medication, past experiences and the relational context. Moreover, individuals who have convinced themselves they are abnormal often experience considerable relief when they learn that desire can follow physical arousal, rather than vice versa.

CAROLINE AND RASHID: A MOTHERING MISMATCH

Caroline and Rashid, both in their thirties, were referred by their GP due to a serious issue in their sex life: whilst Rashid wanted to have sexual intercourse every day, Caroline was content with once a month. During the first session they found it difficult to talk about this intimate subject and it was clear from their body language that the problem was significantly impacting on their relationship as a whole. At home, Rashid was becoming angry and frustrated with Caroline and she was becoming more closed down to his incessant advances.

The therapist discussed how, regardless of age and gender, sexual desire can vary in individuals. They had a young family and Caroline found looking after the children exhausting; she just wanted to be left alone to watch TV in the evenings and have some time to herself. The couple reflected on this with the therapist and also discussed that Rashid felt he was no longer Caroline's top priority. They explored the way in which Rashid communicated his desire for sex – first demanding then sulking when his advances were rejected – and how this placed Caroline in a non-sexual, parental role. His behaviour was certainly not a 'turn on' for her.

> The therapist advised the couple to think about how their individual needs could be communicated better. She also asked them to consider whether they always had to have full sexual intercourse or whether they could do other intimate things that might be less tiring for Caroline.
>
> The couple worked on massages and having showers together. They reported that this began to give Rashid the intimacy he craved and enhanced Caroline's enjoyment as the focus was no longer solely on penetration. They agreed to allocate some time for sexual intimacy at least once a week. During the final session they disclosed that the improved communication and lack of pressure had enabled Caroline to initiate sex for the first time in years.

REFLECT

The fact that Rashid needed sex every day, and his childlike response when he was denied, may have indicated an unmet need for intimacy or comfort as a child. This might explain his behaviour towards Caroline following the birth of his own children. By contrast, for Caroline, the added responsibility of motherhood coupled with her husband's demands left her feeling overloaded and caused her to reject any suggestion of sexual arousal and desire.

RESPOND

Although many sexual problems can be prevented with early intervention, Caroline and Rashid's story illustrates that further referral is sometimes necessary. However, the need for psychosexual therapy should be confirmed with the individual prior to any referral. It is also helpful to share what the therapy sessions might entail and how long they may have to wait. Informed consent to referral builds trust in the engagement both at the time and in the future.

> ### TIRED TIM
>
> At the age of 45, tall and smartly dressed Tim started psychosexual therapy for support in regaining his sexual desire and erectile function. He recalled the death of his wife at the age of 33, and

explained that their children were now young adults who were starting to think about leaving home.

After being in the dating wilderness for many years, Tim was now in an exciting relationship with Becky, who was 13 years his junior. However, while everything had gone well at first, after a while Tim had started to lose his erections during sex. This uncertainty, even with the support of PDE-5 inhibitor medication, had left him feeling tired, which had exacerbated his loss of sexual desire. Indeed, he felt increasingly unable to fulfil Becky's needs for regular and adventurous sex. Tim had experienced no other physical changes and a recent hormone profile was within normal limits for a man of his age.

From Tim's history, the therapist was alerted to issues of loss concerning the death of his much-loved wife and the mother of his children. This seemed important in the context of finding a vibrant new partner with a voracious appetite for sex that over time he could no longer satisfy. The therapy took him through these contrasts and back to a reawakened but previously unspoken grief – the hopeless feeling of being unable to save a woman whose life was 'taken away'. Once the inner conflict and guilt were acknowledged and expressed, Tim was able to see Becky for herself. Although he could not consistently meet all her sexual needs, they entered into a demystified and sexually fulfilling partnership.

REFLECT

The therapist could have explored any number of avenues as to why, in this relationship and at his life stage with teenage children, Tim should have lost his sexual desire, but their sessions together opened up the opportunity to revisit the appalling loss of control he felt on account of his inability to prevent his wife's death. Finally sharing his grief enabled Tim to recover his sexual response and brought him back to life.

RESPOND

In itself, simply giving someone an opportunity to discuss their current or previous circumstances, or what has hurt them the most, can be sufficient to set them on the road to recovery. It also opens the door to effective follow-up.

Gender identity, sexuality and difference in sexual desire   85

Polyamory

Some people strive for the romantic idea of a soulmate, whilst others believe that no one partner can fulfil all of their relationship needs so they prefer to have several at the same time. The practice of forging multiple intimate relationships, whether sexual or just romantic, with the full knowledge and consent of all parties is known as polyamory or 'consensual nonmonogamy' (Psychology Today, n.d.). It is not gender-specific and obviously rejects the idea of exclusivity: a polyamorist feels that anyone can have multiple partners of any gender at any given time. This is different from couples who choose to have casual sex without emotional intimacy with other people. The latter is known as 'swinging' or 'partner swapping'.

RAY, DAVE AND HEIDI: THREE IS NOT ALWAYS A CROWD

Two gay men in their forties – Ray and Dave – attended a clinic for treatment of diagnosed chlamydia. They had been partners since their early teens and the HP smiled as their close connection went as far as wearing identical clothing. Both were baffled as to how they had contracted chlamydia as they stated that they only ever had sex with each other. However, they seemed unperturbed by the diagnosis and accepted the prescribed treatment. At this point the HP stressed that it was their duty to inform any other sexual partners of the diagnosis so they could receive treatment, too.

The following week, a woman named Heidi attended the clinic, handed over a contact tracing card and informed the same HP that she believed she was a contact of someone with chlamydia. The HP noted that the card connected Heidi to one of the gay men. Following a full STI screen, she was prescribed a course of antibiotics. The HP also took Heidi's sexual history and learned that she was heterosexual and had recently had casual sex with a heterosexual male partner. She suggested that the chlamydia must have come from him, but this did not explain the connection with the two gay men. On further discussion, Heidi explained that she lived with Ray and Dave and they had all known each other since college days. A brief relationship with Ray when she was 16 had resulted in a pregnancy, whereupon Ray had disclosed that he loved Dave. By contrast, he explained that his relationship with Heidi had been no more than a brief experiment. Heidi had the baby and they both moved in with the 'boys', where they had continued to live ever since. Ray and Heidi's daughter had never wanted for childcare and she considered both men to be her dads, although she knew that Ray was her biological father. Heidi explained that the boys led their own lives while she had occasional male sexual partners. They were all very happy with the arrangement and it had worked well.

However, the HP still could not understand how Ray and Dave had contracted chlamydia. Heidi explained that she had never stopped loving Ray, the father of her child, and admitted that they still had sex once or twice a year, usually during an overnight stay in a hotel after attending a concert or a theatre show. Moreover, they did not want Dave to feel jealous, so he was always invited to participate in both the excursions and the sex. Heidi said their main concern was that their daughter should not find out, and she conceded that they probably should start to think about living separately at some point. The HP asked her how old her daughter was now and she replied, 'Twenty-six.'

REFLECT

After this consultation, the HP reflected that this was a mutually agreed, long-term relationship between three consenting adults that connected them and their child in a positive way.

RESPOND

This case illustrates that continuous engagement and following up on details not only enables HPs to see the full picture but also increases the likelihood of effective clinical outcomes.

PHILLIPE AND IMKA: FACING TWO WAYS AND MORE

Phillipe and Imka had been in a long-term relationship for several years and were devoted to each other but then Imka started to lose her interest in sex and Phillipe became ever more moody, resorting to childish tantrums when things didn't go his way.

Just prior to their wedding, Phillipe had told Imka that he had previously felt a sexual attraction to – and valued the companionship of – younger men, but Imka was now all he needed. This had reassured Imka and they had proceeded with the wedding. However, since then, Imka had come to accept that one male friend or another would always be an adjunct to their marriage.

Whenever Phillipe started to befriend a new man, he would invariably inform Imka and seek her approval for their sexual liaisons. Understandably, she found this challenging, but she wanted to minimise the risk of him harming himself or their family, so she continued to support him. However, she started to experience regular headaches and exhaustion. Meanwhile, Phillipe had explored the concept of polyamory and tried to convince Imka that this was the best fit for him as it would allow him to nurture the genuine love and affection he felt for the young men.

During therapy, Phillipe began to understand that his wife's lack of sexual desire may have arisen in parallel to his interest in other relationships that had demanded much of his time and attention. However, he had not yet realised that Imka had neither polyamorous nor bisexual desires herself, nor that she had no interest in an 'open marriage'. Furthermore, when the polyamorous relationships failed to meet his expectations, his anxiety and fury would dominate the household, which forced Imka to adopt a soothing, maternal persona.

Phillipe gradually started to recognise that the tensions arising from his sexual choices were putting his marriage at risk. Faced with the very real prospect of losing his children, he started to accept his and Imka's different attitudes towards sex and managed to engage more effectively with her. This gave them the foundation they needed to build a mutually satisfying relationship.

REFLECT

It may be impossible to meet every sexual desire, but many couples manage to negotiate and accommodate each other's needs. Therapy helped Phillipe to identify the source of the tension between himself and Imka and to make a firmer, more adult commitment to his wife's needs, which improved their family life and the nurturing of their children.

RESPOND

It can be hard not to pass judgement on the choices of others. But in this case, yet again, we find that acceptance of an individual's idiosyncrasies can help them to achieve a more satisfying life.

Fetish/paraphilia

When sexual desire and arousal are triggered by an atypical object, fantasy, behaviour or particular kind of individual, animal or body part, this is termed a sexual fetish or paraphilia (Hudson-Allez, 2018). The most common of fetishes are:

- Exhibitionism – revealing the genitals to passers-by without their consent
- Paedophilia – children become objects of sexual arousal
- Voyeurism – looking at others without their consent during intimate moments
- Frotteurism – rubbing against another person without their consent
- Sado-masochism – consensually inflicting and receiving pain for sexual arousal

At one end of the spectrum, a couple might enjoy 'talking dirty' to enhance sexual arousal. Although even this may be considered paraphilic if it becomes the only way of achieving sexual arousal and overrides the relationship. More extreme forms of paraphilia can disrupt life patterns, destroy trust in the self or others and cause significant harm.

The cause of paraphilia remains uncertain, although it may be that a single event during sexual development can unconsciously become a repeated pattern linked to sexual arousal. Paula Hall (2013: p. 1), who has written extensively on the subject of sex addiction, suggests that individuals who are addicted to seeking out a certain form of sexual pleasure that governs their daily activity can be 'imprisoned by behaviours that damage their self-worth and integrity'. This can begin in a gradual way and may be contained within an accepting relationship, but paraphilia can also put individuals at risk of arrest and imprisonment, especially if the activity is non-consensual.

DIMITRI: FEET FIRST

Dimitri, in his mid-forties and with a responsible job, attended for psychosexual therapy, having disclosed to his GP that he had a foot fetish, the nature of which was impacting on his relationship with his partner and child. He attended on his own initially, and when asked about his earliest memory of the fetish described how as a small child he had dropped a toy car in a café. When he bent under the table to retrieve it he saw the feet of a pretty 18-year-old woman and was mesmerised by her brightly painted pink toenails. During puberty the fascination became sexual and he would view women's feet in catalogues and on the street whenever he could.

More recently, Dimitri had visited commercial sex workers who specialised in foot fetish and had used the internet to satisfy his cravings. However, his GP had recently diagnosed him with moderate depression and had prescribed antidepressants.

In the therapy sessions, Dimitri reported that the fetish was out of his control and admitted that he was ashamed of his behaviour. Because of her awareness of Dimitri's low mood and shame, the therapist suggested that they should start work on regaining personal control of the situation, rather than try to stop it all together. He attended the next session with his partner, Sima, who appeared very supportive. Sima accepted that Dimitri was sexually aroused by her feet and they had managed to incorporate this successfully into their love-making. However, in the safety of the therapeutic environment, she disclosed that she felt sad that other parts of her body were not sexually arousing for him. In addition, she was angry at the way he tried to hide his internet use and extremely hurt regarding his visits to the sex worker, from both trust and financial perspectives. There was a lot of discussion around this during the consultation, after which Dimitri acknowledged that this behaviour was unacceptable to his partner, although Sima conceded that his 'extramarital' sexual activity had at least not put her at risk of contracting a sexually transmitted infection.

Dimitri eventually agreed to limit his internet use to scheduled times that he would agree with Sima, and committed not to use a phone that would allow him to access the internet at work. Through this intervention he began to take control of his fetish so that it was no longer in control of him, which enabled the couple to recover their intimacy.

REFLECT

Although on the surface it looked as if the couple had successfully incorporated the fetish into their love-making, Sima's attendance at the consultations gave her an opportunity to be honest about her anger and sadness. In turn, this gave Dimitri the motivation he needed to find a way forward that was acceptable to both of them.

RESPOND

The risk of encouraging patients and their partners to express difficult feelings has to be weighed up carefully. In our experience, sitting back for a moment and listening without taking sides often moves the issue forward in leaps and bounds.

PEEPING TOM

Tom was in his early fifties when he was referred for psychosexual therapy for paraphilia. On collecting him from the clinic's communal waiting room, the therapist was surprised to find him openly reading a book on how to treat paraphilia. When she asked him to sit down in the consulting room, he seemed quite agitated and said, 'I'm not sure I should see a woman. I thought I would be seeing a man.' The therapist asked why this was a concern and he replied, 'Because what I do is to women.' The therapist responded, 'Maybe it's a good thing that I'm female. Let's start the assessment and we can decide later.'

Tom disclosed that he took photos under women's skirts. He would go to London and spend hours waiting for an opportunity. This addiction had contributed to the recent break-up of his marriage, although he and his wife remained good friends. Tom said he desperately wanted to stop this behaviour. He had never been caught but he was worried about his reputation and the impact it would have on his adult children (whom he had told) and his grandchildren if he were to be arrested. His childlike candour was almost charming and he displayed remorse, so the therapist believed that he truly wanted to change.

During therapy, they talked about when Tom's interest first began. He related that he had been fascinated with shop mannequins since about the age of five and would lift up their skirts. Subsequently, around the age of ten, he had watched a pretty teacher in a short skirt running up the stairs and had seen her knickers. This had developed into a sexual fantasy and he would buy photographic magazines for 'peeping Toms'. Later, he had started to take similar photos himself.

After hearing this, the therapist asked Tom to bring in some of his photos. During the next session, she observed a pronounced change in him when he showed her the 'best' ones. Usually shy, quiet and unemotional, he became very animated and excited. When the therapist asked what sort of women he targeted, he said they were always smartly dressed, powerful-looking businesswomen. She asked if he would ever be able to start a conversation with such a woman, to which he replied, 'No, I would never dare. I would be too scared!' This was the therapist's cue to point out that he was being dishonest and deceitful by taking something so intimate from them without their consent. Tom acknowledged this and his shame for doing so. Together they reflected that these women would be unlikely to give Tom a second glance, let alone speak with him, due to their power and class, so the photos were his way of reducing their power and increasing his own.

Tom's therapy concluded after he went 12 months without taking a photo. During the final session, he thanked the therapist and said he was glad he had seen a woman rather than a man.

REFLECT

The female therapist enabled Tom to experience a mutually respectful relationship with a 'powerful' woman. Through this, he found the 'power' he needed to change his behaviour. In addition to Tom's concerns over seeing a female therapist, the therapist had concerns with respect to his presenting behaviours and possible manipulation.

RESPOND

Through the support of clinical case supervision, the therapist was able to stay in role and build a respectful relationship with Tom. Regular, planned clinical supervision enables the therapist to explore any uncomfortable feelings or concerns. Furthermore, sharing concerns with a trusted colleague immediately after an uncomfortable encounter can facilitate deeper understanding of the professional–patient relationship and assist in the maintenance of boundaries. (See Chapter 13 for further explanation.)

Asexuality

Some individuals, such as Amy (see above), have never displayed an interest in sex, nor any desire to engage in a sexual relationship. This does not necessarily mean that emotional intimacy is unimportant to them. It is simply that some people are not naturally inclined to seek out a physical sexual encounter, even with someone they care for. This may be a lifelong phenomenon, but it can be worth exploring, especially if it is causing distress to the individual, their partner, or both (see 'Clive's misconnection' in Chapter 5).

MIA'S MINEFIELD

Mia had never been sexually attracted to anyone, which had left her feeling that she was the odd one out. She was happy in her own company, but longed for close companionship. Was she asexual? The religious community and family culture in which she lived as an adult caused her to feel very low at times, as all close relationships were assumed to be sexual. This added complexity as Mia could not countenance being sexual with anyone. On entering therapy for depression, she was able to share the contradictions of her childhood. Her family were respected members of the community, and the women had designated roles. However, Mia, without a word spoken at the time or since, had endured regular night visits from an uncle who was unable to develop relationships of his own. Her previously silent grief spilled into the safe space of the consulting room.

Thereafter, Mia's low moods became less frequent and she started to enjoy a fulfilling partnership with a very close friend, having first agreed the boundaries of their non-sexual physical intimacy.

REFLECT

The cases in this chapter illustrate that we are ill-advised to make assumptions about sexual practices, sexualities, gender identity or sexual desire.

RESPOND

The first step should always be to give the individual or couple sufficient time and space to describe the reality of their situation. This will enable the therapist to get to the heart of their dilemma with them, offer the appropriate support and identify the best way forward for all concerned.

References

Gurney, K. (2020) *Mind the gap*. London: Headline.
Hall, P. (2013) *Understanding and treating sex addiction*. London: Routledge.
Hudson-Allez, G. (2018) *Infant losses, adult searches: a neural and developmental perspective on psychopathology and sexual offending* (2nd edn). Abingdon: Routledge.
Mitchell, K.R., Wellings, K.A. and Graham, C. (2014) How do men and women define sexual desire and sexual arousal? *Journal of Sex and Marital Therapy*, 40(1), pp. 17–32.
Nagoski, E. (2015) *Come as you are*. London: Scribe.
Paz Galupo, M., Stuart, J.F. and Siegal, D. (2015) Transgender, transsexual, and gender variant individuals, in *International Encyclopedia of the Social and Behavioral Sciences* (2nd edn). Oxford: Elsevier.
Psychology Today (n.d.) Polyamory. Available from: www.psychologytoday.com/intl/basics/polyamory (site accessed 23/11/2020).

Further reading

Berry, D. and Lezos, A.N. (2017) Inclusive sex therapy practices: a qualitative study of techniques sex therapists use when working with diverse sexual populations. *Sexual and Relationship Therapy*, 32(1), pp. 2–21.
Pink Therapy (n.d.) Working with gender, sexuality and relationship diversities. Available from: www.pinktherapy.com (site accessed 23/11/2020).
Science Direct (n.d.) Gender identity. Available from www.sciencedirect.com/topics/social-sciences/gender-identity (site accessed 21/11/2020).

7 Sexual health

Emotions are valued in psychosexual therapy and their expression is encouraged in the safe space of sessions. However, in order to focus on the physical consequences of sexual activity, the risk of emotional and physical harm must be assessed, including the risk of contracting or passing on sexually transmitted infections (STIs). Sexual health across the lifespan is an important part of an individual's wellbeing if their choice is to be sexually active. However, with sexual 'freedom' comes a particular responsibility to self and others. If partners change or sexual encounters are with several partners, regular sexual health screening should be adopted as part of a healthy lifestyle. Psychosexual issues or concerns may be identified in sexual health settings.

We have found that disclosing a personal sexual history, coupled with the anxiety over a potential genital examination, can generate fear. This can be expressed in the clinic through various behaviours, including:

- Avoidance of and non-compliance with testing and treatments
- Tears
- Aggression
- Agitation
- Withdrawal
- Overt friendliness
- Hostility
- Impatience to leave

These reactions may be uncomfortable for the health professional, especially within a busy clinic setting. It can be helpful to acknowledge that some of them may be due to:

- The perceived stigma of attending a sexual health clinic
- The fear of recognition by friends or others

- Concerns over personal confidentiality
- Shame
- Anger and defensiveness due to underlying hurt
- Feeling 'dirty'

It is important to recognise that most people experience these powerful emotions, which can feel overwhelming and hard to control, at one time or another. Acknowledging such feelings can reduce the stress and increase the likelihood of achieving a positive outcome for both the individual and the service providers.

The sexual health consultation

Essential questions of an intimate nature will be asked in the privacy of a sexual health consultation. This is necessary to assess each individual's risk of contracting a sexually transmitted infection (STI) and the test that will be required in order to avoid making assumptions. Effective care in this instance relies on total honesty on the part of the patient, because withholding potentially vital information can lead to further difficulties. In sexual health settings any and all information obtained remains confidential, except in cases where there is serious risk of harm to self or others.

If either the patient or the health professional experiences discomfort during the consultation, this may indicate that something unspoken needs further exploration. Having the confidence to acknowledge these difficult feelings during the consultation can allow shared understanding of any blocks or challenges between the HP and the patient. If such an opportunity is missed by the HP, they will be able to reflect on this confidentially and through clinical supervision. During supervision they can share their professional and personal responses and develop a new perspective on the case, which can be acted upon in further consultations with the patient and/or similar situations in the future.

POOR MAGGIE

Maggie was an emaciated woman who looked older than her 65 years. Attending the clinic for a full sexual health screen, she sat on the edge of her chair, shoulders hunched and head bowed. From the history, the sexual health advisor (SHA) knew that Maggie had recently received treatment for cancer and wanted to understand its

96 *Sexual health*

> impact. Maggie disclosed that a bowel operation had left her with a temporary colostomy and a bag for faecal contents on her lower abdomen.
>
> The SHA assumed that Maggie's grief was due solely to her cancer diagnosis, so she put her pen down and attempted to engage and empathise. With a sudden and angry outburst, Maggie revealed that she felt furious and helpless because the cancer had ravaged her body. Shaking, she explained that no one would want her for sex, which meant she would be unable to sell sex and pay off her debts. She was inconsolable.
>
> The SHA had been unprepared for this additional disclosure, having focused entirely on the cancer diagnosis due to Maggie's frail appearance. On reflection, the shock and discomfort brought to light the health advisor's reasonable assumption that Maggie's fear was related to the diagnosis. However, Maggie's persistent outrage at the effects of the operation revealed a more profound reason for her upset and highlighted the need for a full STI screen.

REFLECT

Even the most experienced professional should never rely on assumptions.

RESPOND

The SHA's encounter with Maggie illustrates the benefits of listening openly with humility and adjusting to the patient's reality. Regular clinical supervision whether in a group or individually supports the HP to grow in understanding and sensitivity whilst learning from others (see Chapter 13 for further details).

> #### TYRONE'S SILENCE
>
> Tyrone was in his thirties when he attended a sexual health clinic. Following tests, he was seen by the SHA to discuss safer sex and condom use. Tyrone was withdrawn and quiet when the SHA began the consultation, which prompted her to ask if he was all right. He began

to describe how awful he had felt during the physical examination with the doctor. He had been given no information, so he didn't know why he was being examined or what the tests were for. The SHA realised that his silence was linked to his shock and discomfort and asked him to go into further detail about how he felt.

REFLECT

Had the uncommunicative encounter with the examining doctor reminded Tyrone of a previous hurtful experience?

RESPOND

It is important for anxiety to be validated as soon as possible as it can affect the perceived or actual quality of an intervention and prevent further unintended harm.

STI screening

Individuals who attend for sexual health screening may experience deep embarrassment and shame, exacerbated by the need for intimate procedures (Heath and White, 2002). Many of the tests in an STI screen can provoke fear and uncertainty, including routine swabs/urine tests for chlamydia, swabs taken from the cervix, urethra, anus or throat for gonorrhoea, and blood tests for Human Immunodeficiency Virus (HIV) and syphilis. Physical examinations to enable clinical observations are performed to diagnose genital herpes, genital warts, Molluscum contagiosum and pubic lice. Further swabs may be taken for Trichomonas vaginalis (TV), bacterial vaginosis (BV), candidiasis (thrush) and Mycoplasma genitalium (MG). Further blood tests may be undertaken for other blood-borne viruses, such as hepatitis B and C. Readers may find more details of some of the signs of STIs on reliable sexual health websites, such as those of the British Association for Sexual Health and HIV and the Sexual Advice Association (see the References at the end of this chapter).

Perhaps surprisingly, many people have a tendency to talk more freely during an intimate genital examination or a blood test. Often the individual may disclose further concerns and may reveal risky sexual behaviour, both of which are likely to heighten the anxiety of receiving the test results. Furthermore, a long wait for the results can exacerbate the apprehension, leading to reactions that may include:

- Deep shock at the discovery of an STI
- Disbelief in a negative result (no STI)
- Blame and anger towards self or others
- Indifference
- Gratitude and increased motivation to self-care

First, it is important to acknowledge that coming forward for testing demands courage. Any of the above reactions on receiving results can provide an opportunity for further discussion as to the implications for that person and their future relationships. It is impossible to predict how someone will react, not least because results that may be considered 'good' for one person may prove challenging for another.

FRANK'S FALL

Frank, a 38-year-old married man with two small children, was pale and anxious when he arrived at the clinic. He disclosed that he had recently had unprotected sexual intercourse with a female colleague during a business trip. He attributed his behaviour to enjoying a brief break from his usual responsibilities and the woman's obvious sexual interest in him.

When the SHA informed Frank that all his tests had come back negative, his response was one of utter disbelief. He was adamant that he must have caught an infection and asked, 'Can't I be treated anyway?' The SHA suggested that Frank's inability to accept the negative results was fuelled by his own sense of guilt and his perceived need to protect his wife. Finally relaxing back into the chair, he said, 'Yes, you're right!'

REFLECT

Frank's fall triggered an unexpected emotion in the HP – exasperation. As the story unfolded, supported by the HPs intuition, we can understand more about this phenomenon. Perhaps she was responding to Frank's own exasperation and his desperation to 'erase' the consequences of his actions? As the HP acknowledged his panic, he calmed down, which enabled him to face his distress and find relief.

RESPOND

Some people return for numerous clinical investigations despite previous negative results and no identified risk factors. This pattern of behaviour can indicate underlying anxiety which may benefit from brief exploration.

AIDAN'S COVER-UP

At the age of 15, Aidan attended the sexual health clinic for a full sexual health screen. The SHA had seen him in the waiting room on several previous occasions, so she double-checked his notes and discovered his results were always negative. She called him into her room for a chat before he went through to see the doctor. Aidan was six feet tall and wearing a brightly coloured puffer jacket. He strode into the SHA's room, took off his jacket and sat down. The SHA observed that he now looked like a young boy. She asked him why he felt he needed another sexual health screen and he said there had been a discharge, indicating his penis. When asked about his sexual relationships he said he had never had sex. On further exploration, it was apparent that the urethral discharge was present each morning when he woke up. The SHA clarified that he was probably experiencing nocturnal emissions (wet dreams) and explained that this was a normal part of sexual development.

REFLECT

The SHA reflected that Aidan had initially appeared 'street wise' and sexually experienced, but in reality he was the exact opposite. The jacket appeared symbolic of his desired strength and confidence, so once it was removed the SHA was able to see his true vulnerability and work effectively with him.

RESPOND

There is value in observing appearance and presentation and how these can change over time. As with Aidan, it may be especially helpful to observe how people present themselves either prior to or at the very beginning of a first consultation. Taking a moment to reflect on words and body posture as well as any mismatch in feeling can support the HP and the patient to identify the heart of the matter more readily.

Human Immunodeficiency Virus (HIV)

HIV is now considered to be a manageable long-term condition due to early treatment reducing the viral load in the body, with life expectancy for those who catch the virus similar to that of comparable, uninfected people. Pre-exposure prophylaxis (PrEP) is readily available in the UK and can be beneficial for many social groups, including men who have sex with men. If taken prior to participating in risky sexual activity, this medication significantly reduces the likelihood of contracting HIV.

However, despite overwhelming evidence that people with HIV are now able to live relatively normal lives, the virus still evokes profound fear and anxiety, underpinned by cultural prejudice and widespread ignorance of medical advances. The following three cases all illustrate the time, patience and understanding that are needed to help others come to terms with their own challenging feelings about HIV.

ANXIOUS ASSIM

Twenty-year-old Assim declared that he would not have sex until after he was married, yet he attended a busy sexual health clinic and urgently requested an HIV test. The SHA saw him to assess his risk. He was panicky and agitated as he explained that he had recently shaken hands with a friend and thought he might have contracted HIV through the sweaty exchange. As he spoke of having several negative HIV tests at other hospitals, the SHA was troubled by his high level of anxiety and fear. Initially, Assim would not be placated despite repeated reassurances that he was at no risk of contracting HIV.

Following this risk assessment, the SHA advised Assim that she would not retest him on the basis of the information he had supplied because the result would again be negative. On hearing this, Assim appeared surprised and speechless. The SHA started to explain the ways in which HIV can be contracted and, as he listened, Assim seemed to absorb this information. He was much calmer when the time came to leave the clinic, and the SHA indicated that he was welcome to arrange another appointment or simply phone for advice should he start to feel overwhelmed again. He took her up on this offer and phoned several times over the next few weeks. The SHA addressed each of his concerns confidently and patiently, and continued to insist that Assim was at no risk of contracting HIV. He eventually stopped calling.

REFLECT

There can be a temptation to offer further clinical investigations in order to reassure patients, but these can be counterproductive as they often feed the original anxiety.

RESPOND

The use of an anxiety scale may help to identify the severity of an anxiety disorder and support appropriate onward referral and treatment.

STUCK SIMON

Simon, in his mid-twenties, had been in a relationship for 18 months and had tested negative for HIV the previous year. Although he was in the same relationship, he requested a further HIV test. The nurse sensed his anxiety as he repeatedly asked the same questions. The nurse asked him why he was so frightened and he confided that he was terrified of contracting HIV. He showed her his reddened sore hands. He had repeatedly scrubbed them in case he had touched anything that might be contaminated with the virus. For this reason, he also used condoms with his girlfriend and was still experiencing rapid ejaculation. The nurse allowed him the time he needed to talk about his fears. When she gave him his negative result he asked to see the paper copy several times. Thereafter, he would ring the clinic every week and ask the nurse to read out the result again.

After several weeks of this, sensing the situation was getting out of control and affecting the couple's sexual relationship, the nurse asked Simon if he would like to speak to a psychosexual therapist. She suggested he might consider inviting his girlfriend along, too.

REFLECT

As is clear from Simon's and Assim's cases, deep fear of contracting HIV can develop into irrational anxiety that affects all aspects of a person's life and relationships.

RESPOND

We should not assume that imparting information and reassurance is sufficient to allay anxiety. An exploration of the source of the fear with each individual may provide more insight. It may also be helpful to ask how the individual is feeling after a negative result. Furthermore, knowledge of local mental health services that can support the patient to work through anxiety issues will ensure that they have some choice in how to move forward and find help.

Following an HIV test within a sexual health clinic, the HP and patient agree on the most appropriate time and manner for delivery of the result – by text, over the phone or face to face. Sometimes the news can generate an unexpected reaction.

PRECIOUS' TIME

Precious, a 35-year-old, smartly dressed woman, arrived at the clinic for her HIV result. Once seated in the consultation room, the SHA informed her that she was HIV positive. On hearing this information, Precious became visibly pale, sweaty and breathless, then ripped off her blouse and bra as if to free her breathing. Although she was unsure of what might happen next, the SHA watched and waited whilst Precious wailed and slid to the floor. The SHA sat quietly alongside her until she had calmed a little, then asked, 'What do you need?' Precious replied tearfully, 'Please can you bring my boyfriend in and will you help me tell him?'

REFLECT

The HP might have been tempted to run away from the situation by leaving the room. However, sitting quietly alongside Precious allowed her to express her extreme distress safely, which in turn enabled the HP to identify the type of support she needed. (See further reflections on Precious' case in Chapter 13.)

RESPOND

When encounters become uncomfortable, it may seem that the best course of action is to walk away or divert to an easier subject. However, remaining present and still, breathing gently in the face of high emotion, greatly reduces the risk of harm. After just a few moments, if asked, the individual will usually be able to articulate what they need next.

Unexpected disclosures of child or adult sexual abuse and assault

Child or adult sexual abuse or past sexual assault can be disclosed at any time and often unexpectedly. Such experiences may remain hidden for decades due to personal shame. Adult sexual function is sometimes – but by no means always – impacted negatively, while sexual desire(s) and fantasies may be altered in some way.

In our experience, a very wide range of childhood experiences – from memories of feeling somewhat uncomfortable during discussions of sex to physical abuse – can disrupt an adult's sex life. Physical abuse encompasses non-consensual sexual touching, exposure to sexually explicit material and partial or full sexual penetration. In all such instances, there is a power differential between the (usually adult) perpetrator and the victim. In addition, a mutually agreed relationship between young people of the same age may deteriorate and become harmful to sexual function. Using personal sexual images against an individual – such as the onward posting of sexting material in the hope of manipulating and shaming the victim – is illegal in the UK. Once again, the perpetrator attempts to seize power and assert control in order to cause harm. This can have an extremely serious, long-term impact on the victim's emotional wellbeing and sexual development.

Any individual who has experienced sexual abuse may live in fear of further exposure. Worry of the unknown and lack of confidence in healthcare professionals may perpetuate their silence. Therefore, the HP should endeavour to acknowledge the impact of such experiences with the individual, highlight any current risk to others and take the most appropriate safeguarding action to challenge and break the cycle of harm.

We have heard victims of sexual abuse offer countless reasons for their previous non-disclosure, including:

- 'It was my fault'
- 'I should have stopped it'
- 'Nobody would have believed me'
- 'I needed to protect others from the same thing'
- 'I was worried what people would think of me'
- 'I was worried what *you* would think of me'
- 'I didn't want anything to happen to my family'

We have also seen the effects of sexual abuse, which are invariably complex and unique to each individual's specific circumstances. As in therapy, it is important to create a safe environment in every consultation as this will encourage the individual to share their disorientating experiences. We have witnessed great courage when people are finally given an opportunity to speak.

Memories of sexual abuse or assault can be triggered unexpectedly in almost any health or social care setting, as the next case study demonstrates.

OLIVIA'S ORAL HISTORY

Olivia, aged 37, dreaded dental appointments but she eventually managed to attend for a check-up with a female dentist, who told her that she required extensive dental work. This evoked feelings of extreme panic, so Olivia asked her GP for help to deal with her anxiety. The GP enquired whether she had ever experienced a similar degree of panic in the past. Olivia was visibly shocked and shaken as she sat back in her chair. She revealed that she had once been flattered by the attentions of a senior male colleague and had invited him back to her flat. However, he had become aggressive, pulled a knife and forced her to perform oral sex on him. She had felt too ashamed and terrified of the consequences to tell anyone.

Following this disclosure, Olivia consented to a psychosexual therapy referral.

Because she now understood the link between the oral sexual assault and the dentist's examination of her mouth, Olivia and her therapist were able to address her suppressed feelings of previously unspeakable outrage. After four sessions of intense psychosexual therapy, she felt she had the necessary confidence to complete the required dental treatment.

REFLECT

Olivia's story may evoke personal or professional memories of similar challenges when delivering or receiving a routine treatment or medical investigation. The assault continued to traumatise her for many years because it remained below the level of her conscious awareness. It was only when an oral examination triggered an attack of debilitating anxiety that Olivia, with the help of a sympathetic GP and a skilled therapist, was able to bring it to consciousness and start to come to terms with it.

RESPOND

Feelings of discomfort in a healthcare consultation can be indicators of previous trauma which may be gently explored with the patient's consent. If the GP had merely offered Olivia a course of anti-anxiety medication, the opportunity for resolution would have been missed and Olivia would have had to face her psychological and physical distress over and over again without ever understanding why.

PAVEL'S BUSINESS TRIP

Pavel, aged 35, was extremely angry, tense and uncomfortable when he arrived at the sexual health clinic. Due to his agitation, he was invited into a quiet room to clarify the cause of his distress. He told the SHA that he had been in a relationship with his girlfriend for approximately ten years and had come to the clinic for a full sexual health screen. The SHA assured him that he was on the doctor's list, but Pavel still seemed agitated. She reflected this back to him and asked him to elaborate on the cause of his discomfort. Pavel revealed that he had been sexually assaulted in the hotel toilets during a business trip. Retrospectively, he now believed that his lager must have been spiked whilst he was relaxing in the bar. The SHA gently asked if he had told anybody about the incident at the time. He angrily replied, 'Oh sure, I came back and told all of my colleagues that I had just been f****** up the arse. What do you think?'

The SHA felt as if she had been slapped in the face. With a sense of shock and shame, she took a deep breath and asked how he felt about the assault now. Pavel admitted feeling despair, anger, shame, loss of control and humiliation.

REFLECT

In this instance the sexual assault was initially disguised by Pavel's anger towards others and silenced by his personal shame at not being sufficiently strong to prevent it. However, the HP understood that Pavel's agitation and anger were expressions of his emotional and physical pain, so she refused to be deflected by her own shame. Instead, she provided the conditions he needed to share his story.

RESPOND

The Survivors UK website (see References) offers personal and professional advice and support for male survivors of sexual assault.

SUBMISSIVE SHEILA

The HP who was explaining the gynaecological procedure that Sheila was due to undergo the following week informed her that she would have to stay in hospital overnight. Sheila went visibly pale, so the HP sought to reassure her that the overnight stay was just a precaution that would enable them to monitor her for 24 hours. However, Sheila still seemed panicky and eventually asked when she would be able to resume having sex. The HP was rather taken aback, but she could sense the seriousness of the enquiry and advised Sheila that it would be between seven and ten days. Still visibly upset, in a very quiet voice, Sheila replied, 'In twenty years I have never had a night away from my husband and he expects to have sex every day.' The HP wanted to say, 'I'm sure he'll understand,' but she managed to stop herself as she suspected he might not.

Sheila's lack of concern for her own welfare and the impending procedure prompted the HP to pass this information on to the nursing team who would be looking after her.

REFLECT

Women like Sheila who are in a domestic violence situation often do not realise that they are also being sexually exploited, as they consent to sexual activity out of fear.

RESPOND

When dealing with individuals who are fully aware of their abusive relationship, it is usually advisable to refer them immediately to safeguarding and support services. However, others need a sensitive, slower approach to gain their trust and further information prior to seeking their consent for a referral.

References

British Association for Sexual Health and HIV (n.d.) Public and patient information. Available from: www.bashh.org/public/public-and-patient-information/ (site accessed 23/11/2020).

Heath, H. and White, I. (2002) *The challenge of sexuality in health care*. Oxford: Blackwell Science Ltd.

Sexual Advice Association (n.d.) Available from: https://sexualadviceassociation.co.uk (site accessed 23/11/2020).

Survivors UK (n.d.) Male rape and sexual abuse support. Available from: www.survivorsuk.org (site accessed 21/11/2020).

Further reading

Department of Health and Social Care (2013) *A framework for sexual health improvement in England*. Available from: www.gov.uk/government/publications/a-framework-for-sexual-health-improvement-in-england (site accessed 21/11/2020).

Jones, R. and Barton, S. Introduction to history taking and principles of sexual health. Available from: https://pmj.bmj.com/content/80/946/444 (site accessed 21/11/2020).

NHS (n.d.) HIV and AIDS. Accessed from: www.nhs.uk/conditions/hiv-and-aids/prevention/ (site accessed 28/11/2020).

NHS (n.d.) Sexual health. Available from: www.nhs.uk/live-well/sexual-health/ (site accessed 23/11/2020).

Rape Crisis England and Wales. Available from: https://rapecrisis.org.uk/ (site accessed 02/02/2021).

8 Women's health

Many people feel understandably uncomfortable with the thought of an intimate physical examination. Once at the clinic, their apprehension and anxiety may manifest in a number of ways, including:

- Little or no conversation
- Lack of eye contact
- Agitation
- Aggression
- Undressing surprisingly quickly or slowly
- Curious positioning of clothing and the modesty sheet
- Refusing to remove relevant underwear
- Closed positioning on the couch

Identifying the feelings associated with an intimate examination at the time can make the procedure more comfortable for everyone involved. In addition, especially if the patient's anxiety is particularly acute, it can help to discuss whether it is appropriate to proceed with the examination on the day or arrange another appointment.

Cervical smear test

In addition to potential anxieties associated with a female intimate examination of the genital area there is the fear of results indicating malignancy and the consequent possibility of invasive treatment. These concerns are sufficient to prevent some women from ever attending a screening. Meanwhile, other women find different reasons to delay or avoid a cervical smear test.

> **TARA'S TESTING TIME**
>
> Following a lengthy discussion, Tara, in her early thirties, finally consented to book a smear test. At the appointment, the nurse asked her to undress from the waist down and lie down on the examination couch. When she returned a few moments later, the nurse found Tara covered with the modesty sheet. However, when she asked her to move her legs into an open position, she was surprised to discover that Tara was still wearing her underwear and tights. It was obvious to the nurse that Tara was so anxious about the examination that she had been unable to follow the clear instructions she had been given. Calmly, she took the time to talk Tara through what would happen during the procedure, which encouraged Tara to remove her underwear and allowed the procedure to take place.

REFLECT

When there is an unnecessary delay in carrying out a procedure, there can be negative consequences for all concerned if the health professional conveys any hint of irritation. In particular, many women recall the negative physical and emotional impacts of insensitively handled and/or rushed intimate examinations. We have found that this can lead to vaginal muscle tightening – known as vaginismus – as an automatic physical response to self-protect from further trauma, a cycle of painful sexual intercourse and consequent loss of sexual desire.

RESPOND

Professional self-awareness of the consequences of insensitive communication during intimate examinations can prevent unintended harm to the individuals in our care. Furthermore, encouraging women to talk through their negative experiences, while refusing to collude in blaming colleagues, as this is invariably counterproductive, can lead to remarkable recoveries.

> **LUCIA'S RELEASE FROM PAIN**
>
> Lucia, in her early fifties, was referred for psychosexual therapy in an effort to resolve a six-year history of painful sex. During the first session, she described a happy, 20-year relationship that had recently deteriorated on account of her inability to have sexual intercourse. The therapist explored with Lucia whether any significant events had happened around the time when the problem had started. The only incident Lucia could recall was a smear test that she had found particularly unpleasant. The therapist asked for further details. As Lucia gave her account tears silently poured down her cheeks, and both she and the therapist were shocked by the power of her distress on recalling the pain and 'coldness' of the examination. Thereafter, Lucia was given the space and time she needed to release her distressed feelings.
>
> Prior to the next scheduled session, three weeks later, Lucia telephoned the therapist to cancel it and all subsequent sessions because her vaginal pain had disappeared and sexual intercourse had become a pleasure again. She was delighted.

REFLECT

It is often impossible to speak out in a moment of trauma, but the body can continue to communicate its distress for many years after. Tara's and Lucia's stories show the importance of monitoring the body's responses during clinical procedures, such as changes in skin colour, hyperventilation, facial tightening and increasing limb tension.

RESPOND

By observing physical responses during intimate examinations, we may be able to prevent the development of psychosexual difficulties.

Colposcopy and hysteroscopy

Further investigations may be required following a cervical smear: for instance, a colposcopy may be suggested in order to take a closer look at the cervix, or a hysteroscopy to look inside the uterus. Again, the prospect of such procedures may generate understandable anxiety and fear. The simple act of acknowledging emotional or physical discomfort can encourage the patient to express their concerns. However, we have learned that excessive reassurance can stifle the truth and prevent further meaningful conversation. (See the Introduction for further information on our therapeutic approach.)

KATIE'S CHANGE OF DIRECTION

Katie was booked for several colposcopies due to the discovery of abnormal cell changes during a routine cervical smear test. However, she cancelled all of the appointments. When she finally found the courage to attend, she was so distressed that the procedure had to be abandoned. The nurse asked why she was so upset, and Katie revealed that the smear test had been excruciatingly painful and she dreaded suffering something similar – or even worse – during the colposcopy. The nurse asked Katie for further details of her experience at the smear test. Katie's face and body changed as she angrily described how the healthcare professional had 'forced' the speculum inside her, leaving her feeling powerless and violated.

The nurse acknowledged Katie's shock and anger while accepting that she could not alter what had happened in the past. However, she was acutely aware that how she responded now could make a big difference to Katie's future. She arranged a new appointment for Katie that allowed plenty of time to discuss the procedure, gave her the option of inserting the speculum herself and made it clear that she was free to call a halt at any time. As a result, both the investigation and the subsequent treatment were successful and conducted with relative ease.

REFLECT

We can all feel very angry when we hear stories of suffering that may lead us to become critical of colleagues. This particular nurse may have been tempted to collude with Katie in expressing her disappointment with other healthcare professionals, but such a reaction may have compounded rather than relieved Katie's distress.

RESPOND

It is important not to be distracted by a patient's anger. Instead, simply acknowledge it, then refocus on their current need for a better experience.

YVETTE'S DISTORTED VIEW

Yvette started psychosexual therapy as she was unable to have penetrative sex. This had begun two years previously, shortly after a colposcopy examination for the treatment of a cervical lesion. The therapist asked her to describe what had happened. Yvette explained that she was frightened of bleeding during sex as she had seen so much blood during the procedure. For the therapist, this description generated a visual image of a huge cervix bleeding profusely. As she reflected inwardly, the therapist offered Yvette a blank sheet of paper and a pen to draw a picture of what she had seen. Yvette drew a huge circle with a large crescent-shaped section, which she indicated was spouting blood.

In light of Yvette's earlier description of her 'huge' cervix and now the sketch, the therapist asked her permission to draw a life-sized cervix on the same page. Yvette was clearly surprised when she saw the second drawing, and recalled that she had viewed her cervix and the blood loss on an electronic monitor during the colposcopy. Together, they realised that seeing this magnified image must have caused her to overestimate both the size of her cervix and the extent of the bleeding. Yvette expressed huge relief as she recognised this. At a subsequent appointment she reported that she had been able to resume sexual intercourse without fear.

REFLECT

If not explained clearly, the language and equipment used by healthcare professionals can generate disturbing images that have the potential to disrupt recovery.

RESPOND

Katie's and Yvette's experiences illustrate the need for clear information as to what to expect of a procedure and the provision of ample time for discussion and feedback.

Further reading

General Medical Council (n.d.). Intimate examinations and chaperones. Available from: www.gmc-uk.org/ethical-guidance/ethical-guidance-for-doctors/intimate-examinations-and-chaperones (site accessed 23/11/2020).

NHS (n.d.) Hysteroscopy Available from: www.nhs.uk/conditions/hysteroscopy/ (site accessed 23/11/2020).

9 Marriage and civil partnership

I thought I was heterosexual
I met her in Greece
I assumed the sun had gone to my head
I had never kissed a girl before.
Back in England, after days, after weeks
I couldn't get her out of my mind.
The weather was miserable, I was miserable.
I had to know, then I knew.
The sun now stays in my heart.
She is my sun.

(Charley Benns, 2019)

Expectations

Many couples are happy to live together without the need for a legally binding contract, but for some marriage or civil partnership is a public statement of commitment, usually involving close family, friends and the wider community. Some dream of that special day and its promise of love, romance and future security. The bond between two people is celebrated and valued by men, women, societies and religions. Instinctively, most believe that it will encompass a fulfilling sexual relationship.

In addition, marriage can hold spiritual significance for religious people. If a couple have abstained from sexual intercourse before marriage, they may have an understandable assumption that sex will be straightforward and rewarding once they are married. Therefore, deep physical and emotional distress can ensue when it fails to meet expectations. Moreover, this sense of failure may develop into an automatic fear response that can completely block the sexual pathway.

In some cultures, the bride to be may receive explicit warnings about the pain and bleeding that she should expect on her wedding night. We have found that such comments can generate so much fear and anxiety that they become self-fulfilling prophecies. Other women may experience an automatic tightening of the band of vaginal muscle (vaginismus) that makes penetration impossible. Equally, a man may be troubled by imagined high expectations of sexual performance, which can lead to 'performance anxiety' and consequent loss of erections (erectile dysfunction; ED) or rapid or premature ejaculation (RE or PE).

Any one of these relatively common problems may cause a couple to avoid sex completely. However, confidential psychosexual therapy can be highly effective in resolving them.

ANITA: BREAKING A FANTASY

Anita, who had entered into an arranged marriage the previous year, attended a gynaecology clinic for an assessment due to a history of non-consummation (inability to have vaginal intercourse). However, the doctor found it impossible to perform an internal examination and asked the assisting nurse chaperone to discuss the matter with Anita.

During the attempted examination, the nurse had noticed Anita's bodily tension and her fearful expression. With Anita still lying on the couch, the nurse asked her why she was so frightened. Anita confided hesitantly that her sister-in-law had told her that sex would be very painful, but she would just have to endure it, as did all new wives on their wedding nights. As the nurse continued to listen, an image of a thick and impenetrable hymen formed in her mind. Then she imagined it tearing and Anita bleeding to death as a result. The nurse waited until Anita had reached a natural conclusion, then tentatively asked if she viewed her hymen in a similar way. Anita admitted that she did, so the nurse encouraged her to place a finger gently into her vagina. Anita agreed, and the nurse asked her to describe what she felt. Anita expressed surprise when she realised her finger entered the vagina with ease. This provided the opening she needed to enjoy a pleasurable consummation of her marriage.

REFLECT

This case study is not intended to give the impression that non-consummation is always due to a fear of pain instilled by a third party. Indeed, there can be many possible causes, and the path to recovery is different for each person. In this instance, the powerful image that came to the HP's mind was certainly unusual, but by sharing it she guided Anita to a successful outcome.

RESPOND

It is important to recognise practice-based experience in the moment, especially if it is unusual. But it is also beneficial to share it in a confidential setting with colleagues as this enables learning from clinical situations to continue. Sharing unexpectedly strong feelings or images with a patient is undoubtedly a bold strategy. If they are not recognised by the patient, then a gentle apology is fitting. That said, more often than not, they will result in further insight and maybe even a crucial breakthrough. Alternatively, it may be advisable to leave especially powerful responses unspoken, but use them to guide the next intervention.

MARK AND MANDY: HURT AND HURTING

Mark and Mandy were a couple in their mid-twenties who had been married for six years. They attended a psychosexual therapy clinic because they found sexual intercourse impossible on account of Mandy's vaginal pain (vaginismus). They had enjoyed sexual activity prior to their wedding, although they had not attempted penetration until after the ceremony.

Mark explained that he had entertained high hopes of the honeymoon and enjoying his first full sexual experience with Mandy. The therapist noticed that Mandy remained quiet while Mark spoke, which led her to ask if she had shared his excitement. In a whisper, Mandy revealed that she had been apprehensive. Looking down, she quietly began to cry and described her sense of failure at letting down Mark. He folded his arms across his chest as he spoke of his deep frustration and disappointment, and disclosed that he no longer tried to initiate sex due to fear of hurting his wife.

Although the couple still enjoyed touching each other, whenever Mark attempted penetration Mandy would push him away as she believed the pain would be unbearable. The therapist remarked that there seemed to be some distance between them.

> They acknowledged this and explained that their relationship had become increasingly argumentative and awkward. Sensing the seriousness of the stalemate, the therapist suggested seeing each of them separately. They happily agreed, and Mark encouraged Mandy to attend first.
>
> During the subsequent one-to-one session, Mandy revealed that she had lost all hope of ever enjoying pain-free sex. Then she mentioned an incident that long predated her relationship with Mark. She had been unable to resist the advances of a man she had known but disliked, which had culminated in unwelcome arousal and vaginal penetration. Following a lengthy discussion, it emerged that anger, distress and guilt had arisen from this experience.
>
> Returning to the present, Mandy asked, 'How come Mark and I were so turned on by each other before we were married? Why has it changed so much?' The therapist suggested that the marriage ceremony opened the door to penetration – a possibility that may have reawakened Mandy's conflicted feelings around the confusing 'disruptive' power of her own and others' sexual desire and her consequent vaginismus.

REFLECT

Unlike Anita, Mandy knew that she was capable of vaginal penetration. However, she feared sexual arousal in herself and others. At a deeper level, she felt that her own arousal would confirm her hidden feelings of shame and guilt. This had led her to question who was really to blame for the teenage assault that had caused her so much profound distress.

RESPOND

Whilst acknowledging that all relationships can be challenging, many couples are able to find a solution if they are prepared to work together. It always seems paradoxical when a couple's long-term relationship breaks down shortly after their decision to make a public commitment to each other. However, as the previous two cases demonstrate, this is precisely when previously hidden personal conflicts often emerge.

GRANT AND SEB: TIED IN KNOTS

Grant and Seb had been in an open relationship for a number of years, but they eventually decided to make a lifelong commitment to care for each other and entered into a civil partnership. They were overwhelmed by the positive responses of family and friends as they celebrated together.

However, after the initial excitement of formalising their relationship, Seb began to avoid sex with Grant. Moreover, on the rare occasions when they tried, he struggled to maintain an erection. As a result, he increasingly looked for sex elsewhere, as he experienced no erectile problems during intercourse with other men. Grant, in turn, was drinking heavily and spending less and less time in Seb's company. He felt low, found it difficult to sleep and eventually started taking antidepressants, which caused him to lose his sexual desire. Unfortunately, neither partner saw fit to raise any of these issues with the other, and within a year they had separated.

Seb related this story several years later, during a routine checkup in a sexual health clinic. Looking back, he recognised that the public commitment had left him feeling trapped and unable to maintain the attraction he had previously felt towards Grant. Indeed, their civil partnership had reminded him of his parents' marriage – precisely the sort of dull relationship that he had always detested. As a result, he had felt an urgent need to escape.

REFLECT

The high expectations of major life events can sometimes end in deep disappointment. In this case, the couple's reluctance to discuss the civil partnership's impact on their relationship meant they had very little chance of increasing their understanding of each other and resolving their difficulties.

RESPOND

Discussing sex can be challenging for any couple, although many would benefit from the involvement of a trusted professional. Therefore, all healthcare professionals should aim to enhance their skills in this area in the interests of improving interactions with service users and securing better outcomes.

Further reading

GOV.UK (2019). Policy paper: marriage and civil partnership in England and Wales. Available from: www.gov.uk/government/publications/marriage-and-civil-partnership-in-england-and-wales (site accessed 29/11/2020).

Hall, K.S.K. and Graham, C.A. (2014) Culturally sensitive sex therapy: the need for shared meanings in the treatment of sexual problems. Available from: https://psycnet.apa.org/record/2014-05878-015 (site accessed 23/11/2020).

10 Hidden loss

Whilst we acknowledge that it can be difficult to discuss the intimate details of sex, it can be even harder to talk about loss. Much of our work involves addressing previously unrecognised loss, and this can be a challenging and painful journey. However, if the timing is right for the patient and they feel safe enough to talk, the release and understanding they experience can bring great physical and emotional rewards.

> **SAFINA AND ABDUL: SEEKING SAFINA**
>
> Safina, in her late teens, was dressed in traditional Indian clothing when she arrived for her first appointment at the local gynaecological department's vaginismus clinic in the hope of addressing the non-consummation of her arranged marriage to Abdul. Her new husband had recently arrived in the UK and spoke very little English. Nevertheless, Safina had encouraged him to attend with her and seemed happy to translate the discussion for him. It soon transpired that the couple had no idea how to have sexual intercourse. With sadness, Safina disclosed that she didn't even know if she had 'a hole for sex'. The HP spent some time explaining basic anatomy, which generated reactions of curiosity and hope.
>
> A month later, Safina attended the next appointment on her own and gave her informed consent to an intimate physical examination with the HP. With guidance and the use of a hand mirror, she was able to see and feel the entrance to her vagina for the first time. She was amazed and delighted by the discovery. Three

months later, she telephoned the HP to cancel her next scheduled appointment as she and Abdul had 'done it' and she was pregnant.

About six months later, the HP was surprised to see Safina on her list of appointments. Heavily pregnant, she gratefully flopped into the chair said, 'I've come back because I've heard you are supposed to enjoy sex but we don't know how!' The HP was happy to explore the ways in which the couple might begin to enjoy their love-making. She also recommended a book of techniques that might enhance their sexual pleasure.

REFLECT

Safina felt the absence of sex in her marriage was a loss to herself, her husband and indeed their whole cultural and religious community. She had clearly received no sex education during her formative years, so it was extremely courageous of her to ask her GP for a referral to a sexual health clinic. As a result, she was able to have sex with her husband and conceive. However, if anything, her decision to return to the clinic towards the end of her pregnancy may have been even more important for her future wellbeing, as it gave her and Abdul the advice they needed to achieve sexual fulfilment. Without that visit, they probably would have continued to suffer in silence, enduring unsatisfactory sex simply to conceive more children and meet their own, familial and community expectations.

RESPOND

Here, as is often the case, the HP's knowledge and sensitivity enabled her to play a critical role in supporting sexual function. As long as the HP listens carefully and identifies the true source of the problem, a subsequent referral can help the patient to take ownership of the next step. A little encouragement to talk about intimate matters often boosts the patient's confidence, which can have a positive impact on both their personal wellbeing and their relationship. This, in turn, may enable them to avoid long-term physical and mental ill-health in the future. Overcoming the impulse to find an immediate solution to problems with intimacy can be liberating for both the HP and the patient.

> **GARY AND ESTHER: GO GARY GO**
>
> Gary and Esther were both single parents, each with three children, when they decided to move in together. At first, they enjoyed a good sex life, but then Gary started to ejaculate increasingly quickly. This left him feeling understandably confused and upset.
>
> As Gary related his story to the psychosexual therapist, his slumped posture and tired voice led her to the conclusion that he was utterly exhausted. When she reflected this back to him, he hurriedly described the chaos of his everyday life since Esther and her children had moved in. He felt that he always needed to be one step ahead to have any chance of keeping up with everything. The therapist suggested that this may be leaving him with few, if any, opportunities to enjoy the present. They discussed how this might be mirrored during sex, as the rapid ejaculation meant that he had finished almost as soon as he had begun, which eliminated any possibility of experiencing sustained pleasure.
>
> It was only when Gary began to talk freely with the therapist that he recognised the enormity of his perceived loss of control as he and Esther tried to juggle the two families. This encouraged him to make some minor changes to their daily routine and free up more time for intimacy.

REFLECT

The rapid ejaculation that Gary experienced spoke of his loss of identity and control within his new relationship and larger family. Once he understood this, he was able to establish a different kind of control that allowed him to restore his and Esther's sexual satisfaction. The psychosexual therapist's recognition of important bodily signals was a key element in this process.

RESPOND

Listening to the body's messages is crucial for health and intimacy. When persistent, undesirable physical changes are explored with an open mind and interpreted in confidence, emotional understanding and physical resolution usually follow.

LIZZIE AND JAMES: LIVING WITH LIZZIE

After ten years of marriage and several failed cycles of in-vitro fertilization (IVF), Lizzie decided to focus on her career and came to terms with the fact that she would never have a child. Then, four years later, at the age of 42, she fell pregnant. The conception obviously came as a massive shock to Lizzie and her husband, James. The midwife at the antenatal clinic and all of the couple's family and friends were thrilled for them. By contrast, deep down, Lizzie felt devastated and out of control. Given the circumstances, though, she was unable to voice these feelings. The couple's sexual intimacy ceased immediately, and 18 months after the birth of their daughter their relationship was so strained that they were contemplating separation.

During psychosexual therapy, Lizzie explored her difficult feelings about raising a child whom she had thought would never exist. She resented her loss of independence and the mundaneness and isolation of caring for a toddler at home while James continued to go to work every day as if nothing had changed. He viewed their daughter as a welcome addition, whereas, for Lizzie, she had come to symbolise the loss of her former life. That said, she never doubted her love for her daughter. Processing her losses over several therapy sessions, Lizzie started to accept both her daughter and her husband, which enabled her to enjoy the new direction her life was taking.

REFLECT

Lizzie felt there was no room for her grief in the midst of her husband's excitement over the unexpected arrival of a baby. As a result, her feelings remained unspoken, which meant they blocked her ability to develop a strong bond with her husband and daughter, leaving her even more resentful and miserable.

RESPOND

We should be more attentive to body language and attitude, in addition to what is said, both during pregnancy and after a baby is born.

Normalising negative postnatal emotions can provide great relief and open the door to further exploration, if necessary.

> ### PETER AND LEO: CATCHING UP WITH DAD
>
> Despite Peter's strong feelings for his new partner, Leo, he struggled to maintain an erection during sex. He had never experienced any sexual difficulties in his previous (short-term) relationships and was distraught.
>
> During Peter's first consultation, the psychosexual therapist asked if he had experienced a similar level of distress at any time in the past. After thinking for a few moments, Peter looked surprised and said, 'I felt just like this when my father died when I was twelve. Endless relatives and friends kept coming to the house to console my mother. I would run off to play with my friends so I didn't have to think about Dad.'
>
> Over subsequent sessions, Peter and the therapist identified a pattern of avoiding difficult feelings, and Peter started to understand the depth of his fear of losing Leo. This led to exploring whether Peter's fear of loss could have undermined his sexual confidence and performance.
>
> Peter had felt a strong impulse to visit his father's grave ever since the first session, but he had continued to put it off, telling himself he was too busy. However, he finally managed to make the trip after several months of therapy. This enabled him to tell his dad about his life and express how much he missed him for the first time. With 23 years of catching-up to do, he took a picnic to the graveside on his next visit. Shortly thereafter, he reported an improvement in his erections.

REFLECT

Peter's early coping mechanism had continued into adulthood, shortening his relationships and blocking emotional connection, until he met Leo. His positive response to therapy shows how a safe professional engagement can facilitate change. In this case, Peter was able to acknowledge that his buried loss and automatic, self-protective defences had been detrimental to his sexual intimacy with the person he loved in adulthood.

RESPOND

It is important to consider the potential impact of a bereavement on every family member. In addition, the loss should be revisited periodically, as people tend to respond in different ways at different times. With patience, this process can facilitate an overall improvement in relationships.

HARRIET: BURYING HER BABY

Harriet, a hospital consultant, organised what should have been a joyful naming and blessing ceremony for her first child. However, on the day itself, she discovered her daughter's lifeless body in her cot. Harriet and her partner had been powerless to prevent their baby's death as she had succumbed to Sudden Infant Death Syndrome (SIDS). Less than a week later, Harriet returned to work and instructed all of the staff never to mention the death of her daughter or enquire how she was feeling. Some of her colleagues were shocked by this injunction, others relieved, but a few were deeply affected as they were unable to acknowledge this overwhelmingly tragic event with her. (See 'Ben's buried loss' in Chapter 1 for a very different response to SIDS.)

REFLECT

Harriet was well aware that she was shutting herself off from the pain of her loss and orchestrating the shutdown of everyone around her. This conspiracy of silence might have helped her to keep functioning professionally, but there is a strong possibility that it also perpetuated her grief and created a block to intimacy.

Responses to grief and loss can be extreme, and delayed grief has the potential to be especially harmful to both the self and others. However, it is wise to remember that not all grief can be immediately expressed through tears and sadness, and some losses are far from obvious, even to loved ones. For instance, we have found that uncharacteristic irritability and anger are often indicators of significant loss. Unspoken grief does not disappear; rather, it tends to grow and may eventually present as physical symptoms.

RESPOND

Making value judgements about a person's reaction to grief is almost always counterproductive, as are unsolicited offers of 'good' advice. That said, everyone who suffers a significant loss, including HPs, should consider taking some time off work in order to begin the recovery process, even if they consider themselves fit to practise and don't want to let their colleagues down.

Further reading

Hackett, M.D., G. et al. (2017) British Society for Sexual Medicine guidelines on the management of erectile dysfunction in men. *Journal of Sexual Medicine*. Available from: www.bssm.org.uk/wp-content/uploads/2018/09/BSSM-ED-guidelines-2018-1.pdf (site accessed 23/11/2020).

NHS (n.d.) Sudden Infant Death Syndrome. Available from: www.nhs.uk/conditions/sudden-infant-death-syndrome-sids/ (site accessed 23/11/2020).

NHS (n.d.) Vaginismus. Available from: www.nhs.uk/conditions/vaginismus/ (site accessed 23/11/2020).

Sexual Advice Association (n.d.) Ejaculation problems. Available from: https://sexualadviceassociation.co.uk/ejaculation-problems/ (site accessed 23/11/2020).

Sexual Advice Association (n.d.) Erectile dysfunction. Available from: https://sexualadviceassociation.co.uk/erectile-dysfunction/ (site accessed 23/11/2020).

Skrine, R. (1997) *Blocks and freedoms in sexual life*. Oxford: Radcliffe.

UK National Institute for Health and Care Excellence (n.d.) Addendum to clinical guideline 37, postnatal care. Available from: www.nice.org.uk/guidance/cg37/evidence/full-guideline-addendum-485782238 (site accessed 23/11/2020).

11 Mid-life

Perceptions of what constitutes 'mid-life' have changed dramatically over recent years. In the 1920s average life expectancy in the UK was in the region of the early to mid-fifties for both men and women, so mid-life was around 30 years of age. Nowadays, the majority of people in Western countries can expect to live to well over 80, so middle age is generally viewed as anywhere between 45 and 60 or even older (Ortiz-Ospina, 2017). We would argue that mid-life is a rather nebulous concept that varies from person to person rather than a set span of years, although the ageing process is always an integral aspect of it.

This stage of life often presents significant physical, emotional and social challenges, but also many opportunities to make a fresh start and enjoy new-found freedom. In either case, sexual health may be compromised, especially as people rarely appreciate the extent to which their lives may change in middle age. Among the issues they may have to face are:

- Unexpected fertility
- Loss of reproductive potential
- Declining physical capability
- A dwindling number of career opportunities
- Menopause
- Andropause (male menopause)
- Attractive daughters
- Competitive sons
- A sudden realisation that time is passing

All of these and many other unanticipated developments can have a dramatic impact not only on how men and women feel about themselves but also on their level of sexual desire.

As in other stages of life, sexual activity can be either enhanced or disturbed by major mid-life events. For instance, when teenagers start to become sexually active, their parents can feel inhibited about their own intimacy. In addition, young people rarely stop to consider their parents' sexual needs, so privacy may become an issue both ways. There is also a general, widespread assumption that sex is unimportant in mid-life. Moreover, for those who have young children in middle age, a combination of fatigue and parental responsibility can have a detrimental impact on sexual desire. That said, we have found that intimacy can be re-established if both partners start to feel heard and appreciated once again.

Some people gain a sense of personal worth from friends, family, partners and others. Social and work roles, along with good health and fitness, can be rewarding, too. On the other hand, if any of these elements are lost or start to decline, problems with sexual function may develop. Unfortunately, both the patient and the HPs they encounter may feel ill-equipped to deal with sexual intimacy issues, with the result that they can be neglected or even completely ignored, especially if the patient is struggling to cope with some of the other challenges of mid-life ageing.

Medical conditions such as raised blood pressure, high cholesterol and reduced hormone levels often develop for the first time in mid-life. All of these can be treated, but the medication may cause or exacerbate problems such as erectile dysfunction, delayed ejaculation and loss of sexual desire. Any such side-effects should be acknowledged and addressed as soon as possible.

Menopause

'Menopause' is the term for women's gradual loss of fertility in middle age, whereas 'perimenopausal' describes the period from the onset of irregular menstruation to when it ceases altogether – years that are often characterised by physical symptoms, such as hot flushes and night sweats, as well as emotional changes, including diminished confidence and heightened anxiety (see NHS, n.d., 'Menopause'). 'Pre-menopause' and 'post-menopause' usually signify the stage before the menstrual cycle becomes irregular and the stage after all menstruation has ceased, respectively.

Some women approaching menopause can start to experience vaginal dryness as well as declines in sexual desire, function and enjoyment. For others, the opposite may be true, as they feel liberated from the possibility of pregnancy. Nevertheless, unwelcome physical changes may still trigger anxiety and ruminations on purpose and value. In addition, the HP might be tempted to treat the symptoms without questioning the impact of prescribed medications on sex and intimacy, not least because sex is rarely considered to be a priority in mid-life.

> **NOT SO SILLY LILLY**
>
> Shortly after starting a new relationship, 55-year-old Lilly visited her GP and requested treatment for vaginal dryness. She was wearing bright, colourful clothes, but she became distraught as soon as the GP pointed out that she seemed tired and pale. When the doctor asked what was troubling her, Lilly looked up and said, 'You are going to think I'm really silly, but I think there must be something seriously wrong with me.' As the GP remained attentive, Lilly went on to explain that sex used to be really easy and exciting, but now, with her new partner, it felt dull. Her doctor suggested some blood tests, just to rule out any possible medical reasons for her loss of desire.
>
> The following week, Lilly's GP reported that the blood tests indicated that she was perimenopausal. In light of this, he discussed the possibility of hormone replacement therapy and suggested a referral for psychosexual therapy to improve her current sexual experience, which Lilly was glad to accept.
>
> During couple counselling, both partners discussed and started to embrace their bodies' changes. With support, they became more sensitive to each other's needs, started using lubrication and initiated sexual experimentation.

REFLECT

As Lilly's wellbeing was important to her, she took the risk of discussing her concerns with her GP. He remained highly attentive throughout the consultation, which left her feeling heard and valued. The referral for psychosexual therapy was especially appreciated, and Lilly walked away from the surgery with her head held a little higher.

RESPOND

This case demonstrates that even the simplest HP actions can make the world of difference to a patient's life. When these actions occur in the context of listening carefully to the patient's concerns, the rewards are not necessarily recognised by either party at the time. However, a subsequent check-in with the patient and taking a moment to acknowledge effective practice can provide the impetus and energy we need to keep delivering patient-focused interventions.

> **LOUISE AND GREG'S NEW CONNECTION**
>
> A middle-aged heterosexual female, Louise, was referred for psychosexual therapy as she was experiencing pain during intercourse. This issue dated back to the start of Louise's menopause, two years earlier. She disclosed that she no longer had any desire because sex was so uncomfortable, and this was affecting her relationship with her partner of 15 years, Greg. She now avoided any physical contact with him in case he became aroused and she could not continue, but this left her feeling guilty, as she knew that Greg missed their sex life. The therapist asked Louise if she missed it, too. She replied that their sex life had been good from the start of their relationship and had remained important to both of them for many years. However, she had felt tired since the onset of menopause, which she attributed to the 'hot flushes' that disturbed her sleep most nights. She also admitted to feeling a sense of loss and sadness due to not being fertile any more. She did not want any more children (both she and Greg had grown-up children from previous relationships), but she still felt she had lost a sense of purpose. The therapist intimated that it was OK to feel what amounted to grief, as this was a significant life stage. Louise replied that she missed being intimate with Greg due to all of these mixed-up feelings, but she did not have the energy to try to fix it. They went on to discuss some of the positive aspects of being more mature – not having to get up early, having more time to reflect and so on – before the therapist concluded the session by suggesting that Louise should consider bringing her partner along next time.
>
> Two weeks later, the couple sat next to each other with their chairs a significant distance apart, and the therapist wondered if this outward display mirrored their relationship. During the session, Greg explained that it was not just the physical act of sexual intercourse that he missed with Louise but simply holding her and smelling her. This had left him feeling lonely. He also stated that he did not want to hurt her and that sex was unenjoyable for him if

she did not enjoy it, too. Finally, he mentioned that he had put on weight and was increasingly fearful of failure, as his erections did not last as long as they had in his younger days. As a result, he was more keen to 'get on with it', but also worried that this might add to Louise's discomfort. At this point, the therapist mentioned that many couples develop a habitual attitude towards sex and arousal in that they are reluctant to diverge from whatever has worked well in the past. However, sometimes the best option is not familiarity but a complete rethink. She suggested that this was an opportune moment for Louise and Greg to discuss what they both liked, needed and wanted from each other sexually. She advised starting with massage, so that they became used to touching each other again, reading a book about arousal and love-making together, then discussing new techniques they may like to try.

At the next session the therapist noted that the couple were sitting much closer to each other, and during their positive feedback Greg took Louise's hand in his and she smiled at him. They reported that they had started to touch each other, but even better was that they had shared their feelings in an atmosphere of mutual support, with no fear of hurt or blame. This new-found honesty and openness had enabled them to become more physically connected and more willing to experiment.

REFLECT

Sexual fulfilment remains possible in mid-life if partners take time to understand each other and adapt positively to their inevitable physical and emotional changes. For women, two of the most common challenges of mid-life are the loss of fertility and the loss of adult children who move away from home. For men, there is the potential challenge of a perceived loss of strength and sexual prowess. However, for both sexes, mid-life can also be a time of transition and reflection during which sexual attraction and intimacy are reaffirmed and even enhanced.

RESPOND

We all know that change is impossible if we insist on doing the same things over and over again. Louise and Greg eventually achieved the change they wanted because they discussed their problems and agreed on the best way forward. This was their greatest breakthrough. It is always worth making the time to talk through any desire for change in an atmosphere of mutual respect and openness.

Andropause

The term 'male menopause' – or 'andropause' – is used to describe the stage of life when men start to produce lower levels of a number of important hormones. This can cause trouble sleeping, fat redistribution around the abdomen and breast area and loss of muscle mass, all of which may be reflected in declining energy, physical weakness, lethargy, low mood and a lack of motivation (NHS, n.d., 'Male menopause'). Some men also lose all interest in sex, while others retain a keen interest but have trouble maintaining an erection. Either condition can be extremely distressing.

Testosterone is an important hormone for all human beings, although, as with so many hormonal and nerve connections between the brain and body, as well as internal and external triggers of physical changes and the ageing process, we still know relatively little about it. That said, there are some effective medical treatments for 'late onset hypogonadism' (reduced production of testosterone), and lifestyle changes can make a significant difference, too. Moreover, some men never experience the andropause and continue to have fully functioning reproductive organs throughout their lives (Healthline, n.d.).

Here, it is worth noting that Greg (in the previous case study) displayed at least two of classic signs of andropause – weight gain and some difficulty maintaining an erection – that may have warranted further exploration. However, in his and Louise's case, greater candour and a willingness to experiment proved sufficient to turn the tide in the right direction. During psychosexual therapy, all options should be considered in the interests of restoring sexual function. And consultation with the primary physician may be necessary further down the line if, for instance, erectile dysfunction remains an issue.

DIRECTING DEREK

By the age of 56, Derek no longer looked forward to sex, nor to exercising or even leaving the house. This was all in marked contrast to his earlier years, when he had enjoyed a good sex life and lots of physical activity. Now, it was all he could do to put in a full day's work, watch TV in the evening, go to bed and start all over again the next morning. He hadn't had a good night's sleep for years. He felt low and useless. He had put on weight and developed what he called 'man-boobs', which made him feel unattractive. His long-term partner was irritable and so was he.

Nevertheless, Derek would often joke about his body and his lifestyle. Eventually, one of his friends grew concerned and directed Derek to consult his GP. This was the push he needed, and after a brief consultation he was referred to the local talking therapy service for help with his low mood. In addition, blood tests were taken to diagnose and treat any underlying medical issues. He was also advised to eat healthier, cut down on the takeaways and drink less alcohol.

After a few weeks of therapy, Derek admitted that he would feel much happier if his sex life could be sorted out. As a result, he was referred for psychosexual therapy, during which the therapist immediately recognised that he was exhibiting two of the classic signs of andropause: his nights were disrupted by sleep apnoea and worries about work kept him awake into the early hours. Thereafter, Derek revealed that he had lost much of his confidence, self-worth, virility and sense of purpose over the previous four or five years. He and the therapist also explored ways of bridging the physical and emotional divide that had grown between himself and his partner.

Derek gained a deeper understanding of everything that may have contributed to his loss of sexual desire, took medication for his low testosterone and improved his diet. These changes enabled him to regain much of his former confidence, and his relationships with himself, his partner and others all started to improve.

RESPOND

Many men find it hard to discuss their personal concerns seriously, but their apparently light-hearted, self-deprecating banter may indicate that all is not well. In such circumstances, they may need no more than the sensitive suggestion of a medical check-up to start their journey to better health and wellbeing (Sexual Advice Association, n.d.).

In mid-life, sexual dissatisfaction within a long-term relationship may lead to infidelity in the hope of achieving greater sexual connection with a new partner. This urge can be especially strong among those who start to identify as gender non-binary or embrace a different sexual orientation in middle age. Other people worry that something is wrong with them following the loss of sexual desire, so they look elsewhere simply to explore whether they can still function sexually. While this may provide temporary reassurance, it usually fails to address any relationship or contextual issues that may have contributed to the problem in the first place; indeed, it is likely to damage or even destroy the long-term relationship should the partner find out. That said, Damien's case highlights the importance of resisting the temptation to make assumptions about arousal outside a valued relationship.

DAMIEN: PAST, PRESENT AND FUTURE

Damien, a 49-year-old married man, attended a sexual health clinic for help with his increasing difficulty in maintaining an erection during sex with his wife. Then he shyly revealed to the sexual health advisor (SHA) that he had been propositioned by two attractive young women during a night out with friends. This had surprised and delighted him, and had resulted in an unexpected erection. However, he was shocked by his sexual arousal as being a faithful husband and a loving father had always been an important part of his self-identity. The SHA asked for more information about his marriage and Damien revealed that he 'worshipped' his wife even though she had never really returned his affections. Indeed, until recently, their only closeness had been through sexual contact, which was why he was so dismayed at his loss of function and his unexpected arousal towards the two young women.

Damien's inability to experience the intimacy of sex with his wife had allowed him to realise how little she gave him. This, coupled with her frequent complaints and criticism, had generated overwhelming but previously hidden feelings of anger and sadness. When the SHA asked if Damien had experienced similar feelings in the past, after a moment he recalled an almost identical reaction to his father's constant criticism and violence during his childhood. In the present, these powerful emotions had rendered him impotent, but a little unexpected interest from a couple of strangers had been sufficient to bring him back to life.

REFLECT

In the past, Damien had tried to protect his wife by suppressing his anger and sadness at the way their relationship had developed. This may have reflected his determination not to behave like his bullying father. However, unsurprisingly, over time, it proved to be detrimental to their sexual intimacy. By avoiding all potentially challenging communication, Damien lost the ability to express his true emotions. In order to protect himself, his body had 'downed tools' (given up) by failing to maintain an erection. However, by discussing the incident with the two women during therapy, he realised that full sexual function and a more honest marital relationship were both within reach.

RESPOND

Who is brave enough to talk about sexual difficulties in mid-life? Who will sensitively encourage acknowledgement of the possible impacts of major life events and illness on sex and intimacy? This is an important aspect of any intervention that seeks to enhance health and wellbeing. However, once the invitation has been made to explore the impact of relevant life events, the patient should always retain the right to share their experiences or not, depending on their particular circumstances and sense of safety.

Surgery and medical conditions

We have already outlined some of the many natural responses to invasive surgery, medical treatment or new diagnoses, such as diabetes. In particular, life-threatening conditions, as well as the associated fear of dying and facing personal mortality, may lead to unexpressed distress. Moreover, guilt about the physical after-effects of treatment or denial of the loss that is frequently felt when the body has been changed by surgery may disrupt intimacy. Finally, difficult emotions such as anger, grief and pain may be left unspoken due to a sense of shame that one should feel nothing but gratitude after a successful medical intervention. However, it is important to acknowledge such emotions, as this will allow the patient to adapt to the physical – and sometimes, but not always, sexual – consequences of their medical treatment.

As we have seen many times in our practice, although most patients are more than happy to accept the physical and emotional support they receive in the immediate aftermath of surgery or other serious medical treatment, they are often reluctant to seek help for issues that emerge later. Websites may prove useful in this respect, as they can offer information, advice and support for those who are struggling to cope with life-changing ill-health (e.g., Cancer.net, 2018; Crohn's and Colitis UK, n.d.; Diabetes.co.uk, n.d.). There are also many nation-specific online support groups.

Eileen's story, below, illustrates the importance of recognising grief and reopening the door to honest communication with loved ones.

EILEEN RISING

Eileen, in her mid-fifties, was referred for psychosexual therapy by her GP following a right-sided mastectomy as she was struggling to cope with the surgery's impact on both herself and her relationship with her husband. Sitting in front of the therapist for the first time, she described her fear prior to the operation as well as a number of traumatic experiences during chemotherapy: on one occasion she had nearly stopped breathing and on another she had suffered such an extreme reaction that she had been hospitalised for five days.

Over the course of the next few sessions, Eileen explained that she had been a confident woman who had enjoyed life as a professional stage performer, but she now felt unattractive and hated her 'mutilated' body. As a result, she had lost much of her confidence. Even buying a dress or a top was distressing as her right arm was larger than her left, which made it difficult to find suitable sleeves. Moreover, her despair was compounded by a sense of guilt whenever she experienced a negative emotion, as she knew she was lucky to be alive. She had been offered reconstructive surgery but did not want to burden the NHS any further and did not know if she could face further surgery. Nevertheless, the therapist explored this subject several times with her to ensure that she understood it was still an option.

Eileen described how her husband of 16 years had been incredibly supportive and kind. However, she also disclosed that they had not been intimate for 18 months – ever since the operation. She now undressed in the bathroom as she was terrified of him seeing her scar and reacting with repulsion – a potential response that would have mirrored her own. Prior to the operation, they had both enjoyed their sex life, having sex at least once a week, but she explained that this was simply not an option now.

Having already worked on the personal trauma that resulted from Eileen's cancer diagnosis and treatment, the therapist realised that the 'disease' had actually affected every aspect of her life and that she was experiencing enormous grief. She suggested that Eileen should invite her husband to attend the next session as it would be helpful to hear his thoughts on the situation.

During the subsequent, highly emotional session (for both the couple and the therapist), Eileen's husband described how much he loved her and explained that he was immensely proud of her, especially in light of all she had recently endured. He admitted that he missed the woman she used to be and really missed being physically intimate with her, but he was terrified that any sort of approach might upset her. At that point, Eileen reiterated that the scar was disgusting and said she was ashamed of her body. Her husband replied that he had seen it in the mirror, and he didn't find it disgusting. It was still her body and he loved her just as much as he had before. It was obvious that they had both been trying to protect each other by suppressing their feelings. They cried and hugged each other, and Eileen agreed to show her husband the scar when they were alone together.

Eileen arrived for her final session fully made-up and wearing a brightly coloured blouse. She disclosed that she and her husband had enjoyed some sexual contact and cheerfully announced that she had bought a very expensive swimming costume in preparation for their upcoming holiday. She was confident that they would soon feel sufficiently comfortable with each other to resume intercourse. In addition, she insisted that she did not need reconstructive surgery, as she had already got her life back. As Eileen walked out of the door, the therapist pictured her taking to the stage again.

REFLECT

In addition to altering the patient's body, invasive cancer treatment can have a profound effect on their partners and their intimate relationships. Eileen and her husband had endured 18 months of unshared feelings and consequent misunderstandings. However, their intimacy returned shortly after they received the support they needed to discuss the 'unspeakable'.

RESPOND

HPs need to be aware of the significant impact of a cancer diagnosis and subsequent treatment. It is important to discuss all of the possible consequences in terms of altered body image, sexual intimacy, desire and relationships as this can lead to improvements in the patient's quality of life and help them to regain a 'sense of normality'.

> Joseph, a 55-year-old man of Afro-Caribbean heritage with a lively sex life, received a late diagnosis of prostate cancer. His condition required radical surgery in order to save his life. On a surgical follow-up appointment, he asked the surgeon whether he would be able to have sex again. The surgeon told him that would be extremely unlikely, then left the room with an air of professional satisfaction that the operation had been a success. Joseph, by contrast, was plunged into a state of shock and desolation by the revelation. He turned to the nurse and said, 'If I had known that I wouldn't be able to have sex again, I never would have agreed to that operation. I'd rather be dead!' The nurse offered a specialist follow-up, which Joseph gratefully accepted.

REFLECT

Whilst the operation may have saved Joseph's life, his pride in his sexual potency was a central aspect of his personal identity. His powerful reaction to the surgeon's news reflected not only this but also a lack of preparedness for the possible consequences of surgery. Moreover, his despair was compounded by the surgeon's casual attitude and disinclination to offer further support and guidance.

RESPOND

All aspects of the patient's personal and cultural context should be considered prior to any treatment, especially when it may impact on their sexual function. In such cases, specialist counselling should always be offered.

Losses and gains

Any loss can have a significant impact on sexual behaviour and/or function. Sometimes serious medical conditions, such as coronary heart disease or cancer, trigger an increase in sexual desire as an affirmation of being alive. Equally, they may result in complete disinterest in sexual activity, or irrational fears that it could jeopardise the treatment. Moreover, a partner's sexual responsiveness may change during challenging periods of ill-health. In such cases, every effort should be made to hear and understand both partners' perspectives.

> **ALAN'S SEARCH**
>
> Alan was an overweight man in his early fifties who presented at a sexual health clinic and hesitantly requested a consultation. He told the SHA that he had experienced a 'massive heart attack' six months earlier, then talked at length about the consequences, showing his scar and the array of tablets that he took each day. Finally, he came to the point of his visit: could he still have sex? The SHA told him she admired his courage for walking into a sexual health clinic and asking that question, but inwardly wondered why nobody had thought to explain the situation to him previously.
>
> Alan continued that he had been fit and active prior to the operation, but the severity of his condition had forced him to give up the job he loved – caring for people with physical disabilities. Consequently, he had lost contact with his former colleagues, and his wife had increased her working hours due to the couple's financial difficulties. He became quite upset when he described how his children treated him like a child and admitted to feeling utterly useless. The only time he felt truly alive was when he was playing with his young grandson, who treated him just as he had prior to the illness.
>
> Alan and his wife wanted to be intimate with each other, but they rarely attempted intercourse as he had been unable to maintain an erection since the operation. He confided that whenever they did try, he was terrified that he might suffer another heart attack. The SHA realised that Alan had not shared this fear with his wife, so it was blocking their intimacy. She reflected this back to Alan, which prompted him to express his overwhelming sadness at the perceived loss of his manhood as well as his supposed diminished status within his family and the wider community.

REFLECT

An unexpected life-threatening episode can lead to a profound loss of confidence and diminished wellbeing. Although there is usually an initial outpouring of gratitude and relief that one has survived, this is often followed by greater appreciation and acceptance of the fragility of life. In turn, this may lead to serious doubts about relationships, physical capabilities and sexual performance as well as an overwhelming fear of death. Moreover, family members will likely experience their own potential loss – or fear of loss – and will also need to process these feelings.

RESPOND

It is valuable to notice what helps and what hinders recovery for the patient. Alan's family were understandably protective (see Figure 0.2 in the Introduction), but this left him feeling useless. Instead, we advocate our 'Therapeutic Space' approach (Figure 0.3 in the Introduction), which allows personal autonomy to return.

GLORIA'S GAIN

A physiotherapist referred 48-year-old Gloria for psychosexual therapy following pelvic-floor treatment for an 18-month history of painful sex. The therapist noticed that Gloria seemed embarrassed and uncomfortable as they started the first session. She spoke quietly and voiced her concerns about wasting the therapist's time. However, when asked if anything significant had happened during the previous 18 months, Gloria bravely spoke of her 30-year-old daughter's diagnosis of breast cancer, subsequent mastectomy and eventual death.

The therapist encouraged Gloria to share her grief, which led to more questions about how it had affected her relationship with her husband and their sexual intimacy. Gloria grimaced and admitted that she could no longer bear her husband touching her breasts during foreplay; she would physically recoil from him if this started to give her any pleasure. This response was clearly linked to her daughter's breast cancer and to memories of how she had fed her as a baby, as both the therapist and Gloria herself acknowledged.

Gloria's repulsion during foreplay had prompted her and her husband to move rapidly to vaginal penetration, with the inevitable result that this was dry and painful. The therapist asked if she might be angry with her husband. Gloria seemed shocked at the suggestion and assured the therapist that the loss of their daughter had actually brought them closer together. She began to cry quietly as she talked of her guilt and sense of injustice that she had breasts and was still alive. This led to a realisation that she may have been denying herself sexual pleasure because of the nature of her loss.

After acknowledging her feelings, Gloria was able to rebuild her sexual relationship with her husband as they found solace in each other and the strength to cope with their mutual grief over the death of a much-loved daughter.

REFLECT

Alan and Gloria both suffered unexpected losses. Alan's manhood and self-worth were profoundly undermined by his heart attack, which also impacted on how others viewed him. His sole link to normality was his grandson, who treated him no differently.

Gloria lost the ability to mother, nurture and, ultimately, save her child with the result that she could no longer experience any joy in her own femininity. She finally found solace in the shared grief, emotional strength and physical intimacy of her relationship with her husband.

RESPOND

Alan's and Gloria's cases illustrate the value of further exploration of emotional context whenever someone presents with a physical dysfunction in order to shed light on any unique precipitating factors and their consequences for personal wellbeing. We have found that this sort of intervention often supports full recovery.

WIDOWED WENDY

From the outset, the therapist sensed that 62-year-old Wendy felt uncomfortable. Her history stated that she had been widowed ten years previously but had recently remarried. However, she was finding sex with her new husband difficult. The therapist carefully encouraged Wendy to explain the precise nature of the problem.

She became tearful and disclosed that her sex life had been good with her first husband, but now it was just not working and she felt a failure. The therapist realised that Wendy was trying to replicate her earlier positive sexual experiences with her new husband, so she reassured her that most couples who have been together for a long time develop a comfortable sexual routine, but subsequent partners may respond to arousal in different ways. Wendy seemed to accept this, but then admitted to experiencing guilt about being with someone else as well as disappointment because, no matter how hard she tried, she could not experience arousal or pleasure during sex. The therapist found this description of Wendy's awkwardness in the bedroom uncomfortable, which she reflected back to her. After this, Wendy revealed that her new husband had told her that he was not enjoying their sex life, either.

During her third and final session, Wendy sat in the chair with an air of renewed confidence and informed the therapist that she had discussed her lack of confidence with her husband. This had given both of them the licence they needed to share their sexual preferences. A few weeks later, Wendy reported back that she and her husband were enjoying greater intimacy and sexual pleasure.

REFLECT

This was a new, exciting phase in Wendy's life, following the loss of her first husband. However, when she found sex with her new husband unfulfilling, especially in comparison with what she had experienced previously, she lacked the confidence to tell him anything was wrong. This challenging situation illustrates that sexual intimacy is more than just a physical response; establishing a strong emotional connection is equally vital.

RESPOND

Both Wendy and her second husband drew on their previous sexual experiences without any discussion of each other's preferences. As a result, both were left unsatisfied by their sex life. This served as a useful reminder to the HP not to make assumptions or focus purely on physical symptoms.

References

Cancer.net (2018) Side effects of surgery. Available from: www.cancer.net/navigating-cancer-care/how-cancer-treated/surgery/side-effects-surgery (site accessed 05/02/2021).

Crohn's and Colitis UK (n.d.) Support for you. Available from: www.crohnsandcolitis.org.uk/support (site accessed 05/02/2021).

Diabetes.co.uk (n.d.) Welcome to the global diabetes community. Available from: www.diabetes.co.uk (site accessed 05/02/2021).

Healthline (n.d.) What is male menopause? Available from: www.healthline.com/health/menopause/male (site accessed 24/11/2020).

NHS (n.d.) Male menopause. Available from: www.nhs.uk/conditions/male-menopause/ (site accessed 23/11/2020).

NHS (n.d.) Menopause. Available from: www.nhs.uk/conditions/menopause/ (site accessed 23/11/2020).

Ortiz-Ospina, E. (2017) 'Life expectancy': what does this actually mean? Available from: https://ourworldindata.org/life-expectancy-how-is-it-calculated-and-how-should-it-be-interpreted (site accessed 23/11/2020).

Sexual Advice Association. Available from: www.sexualadviceassociation.co.uk (site accessed 23/11/2020).

Further reading

Age UK (n.d.) Sex in later life. Available from: www.ageuk.org.uk/information-advice/health-wellbeing/relationships-family/sex-in-later-life/ (site accessed 22/02/2021).

Beddington, E. (2020) The truth about midlife dating and sex. *Sunday Times*. Available from: www.thetimes.co.uk/article/the-midlife-guide-to-dating-and-sex-rlf00tp50 (site accessed 24/11/2020).

Help Guide (n.d.) Better sex as you age. Available from: www.helpguide.org/articles/alzheimers-dementia-aging/better-sex-as-you-age.htm (site accessed 24/11/2020).

Lewis, R. *et al.* (2019) Navigating new sexual partnerships in midlife: a socioecological perspective on factors shaping STI risk perceptions and practices. *Sexually Transmitted Infections*. Available from: https://sti.bmj.com/content/sextrans/early/2020/02/09/sextrans-2019-054205.full.pdf (site accessed 24/11/2020).

Menopause Matters. Available from: www.menopausematters.co.uk (site accessed 24/11/2020).

12 Older age

> Old age is a bugger isn't it?
> (Sir Frederick Ashton, British choreographer, aged 82, private family correspondence)

Adapting to later life

For many, life comes full circle in older age as aunts, uncles and grandparents witness the lives of subsequent generations playing out differently or similarly to their own. From the excitement of a young couple getting to know each other to travelling on life's journey together, the challenges of maintaining intimacy continue into older age. This can present opportunities for the couple or it may be a challenging and awkward time as they struggle to adjust to the physical and emotional changes that are inevitable aspects of the ageing process.

> ### BERYL'S BRAVERY
>
> Beryl, in her late seventies, attended a gynae outpatient clinic as her vaginal ring pessary was due to be changed. The nurse was just about to invite her onto the examination couch when Beryl told the doctor that she was keen to know about other treatment options for her pelvic organ prolapse. He asked if she was having problems with the ring pessary and seemed visibly shocked when Beryl said that it was doing the job well, but her husband found it uncomfortable when they had sex. With a laugh, Beryl said, 'You look surprised. Of course, we don't do it as often as we did when we were younger, but we still enjoy having a bit of fun every now and then!'

FRAMED FREDA

The HP read the referral letter prior to seeing her next patient in a specialist gynaecology clinic for women with vaginismus. It stated that the woman, in her early seventies, had recently had a vaginal repair and wanted confirmation that her vagina had returned to normal. It went on to say that sexual intercourse would 'obviously' not be an issue for her. The HP was irritated by that assumption as she went to call Freda from the waiting room. Freda stood up with her elderly husband and walked into the consulting room with the aid of a walking frame, which prompted some amused glances from the other nursing staff.

During the consultation, the HP asked Freda if she wanted to have sexual intercourse now that she had recovered from the operation. Freda replied, 'I'm not too worried but you would like to, wouldn't you Albert?' He replied that he would and they both smiled. The HP examined Freda and advised that the couple could have intercourse as she had not experienced any pain throughout the examination. As the couple happily left the clinic, one of the nurses commented to the HP, 'Surely they weren't in your clinic, were they?' The HP replied firmly, 'Yes, they were, and they want to continue to have sex.'

REFLECT

Enjoyable sex was still a very important aspect of Beryl's and Freda's lives. Beryl was able to make light of the shocked look on the doctor's face, but other women may have been reluctant to talk about their sex lives with such candour. It is also worth noting that even health professionals can make incorrect assumptions that older people no longer enjoy sexual intimacy, as the nurses' reaction in Freda's case illustrates.

RESPOND

It is vital to consider that many patients in their golden years continue to enjoy sexual intimacy, as this is relevant to their healthcare. Beryl's and Freda's cases demonstrate that questions about sexual function are usually welcomed as long as they are relevant to the healthcare intervention.

New challenges in old age

New sexual relationships may develop in older age, such as after the loss of a long-term partner. Although sexual activity with a new partner can be exciting, it can also present challenges. For instance, the fear of comparisons with previous partners and high self-expectations can lead to disappointment as well as feelings of failure and isolation. On the other hand, the experience that comes with older age can give sexual partners the confidence they need to express their preferences freely. That said, for some people, the thought of any form of intimacy with another person after the loss of a partner is simply unacceptable. For others, coping with the physical changes of older age may require inventive approaches to making sex more comfortable, especially if one partner has become the other's carer. In such cases, it is important to consider that attitudes towards sex may change, too. Professional help is available for older people who wish to explore other expressions of intimacy in addition to sexual intercourse.

REGGIE LETS HIMSELF OUT

Reggie, in his mid-seventies, attended a sexual health clinic complaining of a discharge from his penis. Following a full sexual health screen, he was prescribed medication for gonorrhoea and chlamydia. In the course of the consultation, as Reggie gave animated descriptions of his recent sexual encounters, the sexual health advisor felt as if she were listening to a teenager. She requested more information, and Reggie revealed that he had gradually recognised his sexual preference for men as he and his wife had raised their children. However, he had not disclosed this to anyone nor acted on his feelings out of respect for his family and a determination not to hurt them.

However, following his wife's death, despite his grief, Reggie had granted himself permission to explore his sexuality without fear or constraint. He had enthusiastically made sexual contacts through the internet and had invited several men to his home. He appeared to have no understanding of the risks that this sort of behaviour posed to his health and safety. The SHA concluded the consultation with a brief but crucial lesson on the basics of self-protection and safer sex.

REFLECT

The thrill of entering a world that he had previously only dreamed of, together with his eagerness to make up for lost time, meant that Reggie gave no consideration to his personal safety. Once this was acknowledged, the risks could be addressed. Sexual health statistics show significant increases in both the number of sexual partners and the prevalence of STIs among older people, probably due to changes in personal circumstances later in life and widespread access to online dating (National Institute on Aging, n.d.).

RESPOND

Maintaining open-minded respect for the patient is paramount in order to gain an honest account of their sexual activity. Without this information, it is almost impossible to facilitate informed choices, prescribe effective interventions or ensure treatment compliance.

MISS G AND EDITH: TOUCHED BY MISS G

At the age of 73, Miss G was being seen by her practice nurse for repeat antidepressant medication following the death of her partner, Edith. However, the nurse found engagement difficult, as Miss G was very reserved. During one of the appointments, as Miss G talked about Edith with her usual lack of emotion, the nurse looked carefully for any sign of grief. She noticed that Miss G would stroke her left breast whenever she mentioned Edith's name. The nurse shared this observation with Miss G, who was immediately taken aback. She recalled that Edith had tenderly stroked her left breast before they went to sleep each night, then wept as she finally acknowledged the deep loss of physical closeness she had experienced due to Edith's death.

REFLECT

Miss G and Edith had engaged in a lifelong, intimate but clandestine relationship, and this seemed to extend into Miss G's locked-in grief response.

RESPOND

When engagement with a patient is unusually difficult, it may be helpful to sensitively persist in exploring the reason why.

Realities of sexual activity in later life

Below, we present an extract from *Doing Anything after Work ... What about Retirement?*, a collection of older people's personal experiences, including physical and emotional intimacy:

> After all this freedom the arthritis in my hands and wrists began to get worse. Who can have really enjoyable sex without using your hands as well as your body? I felt a bit resentful, but was firmly told that this is the way it is when you get older. Gradually I got used to the discomfort and the arthritis decreased slightly as time went on. But then a worse thing happened. My partner went to the GP with a minor complaint. The GP decided to take his blood pressure. It was up, so drugs were prescribed. Exactly two weeks later he started having problems with sex never having had any difficulties before. Change of drugs made no difference.
>
> I felt cross that the GP prescribed NHS Viagra to men of sixty but not for my partner who was well over seventy. This was a real case of ageism. However, when we tried over the counter Viagra, it wasn't much good anyway for drug induced symptoms. Then in a real moment of love and consideration he went into a sex shop with great embarrassment and brought me a present of a silver friend with a battery. In mutual sex it gave me fantastic climaxes, which we both enjoyed. Now we are both a bit older, bodily contact and snuggling up are both very enjoyable but the full works is much less often and we accept this.
>
> (Anonymous contributor quoted in Bramley, 2009: p. 64)

Couples who manage to work through and accept their physical limitations after retirement, and those who grieve for their losses, often enjoy enhanced physical and emotional intimacy later in life. For some, such as Reggie (see above), the loss of a long-term partner may liberate previously suppressed sexual longings and allow their full expression for the first time. It is important to remember that the sexual health needs of older people require as much care and attention as those of younger people (see Age UK, n.d. for further information).

In *Being Mortal*, Atul Gawande illustrates the importance of intimacy in older age and ill-health with reference to a couple named Bella and Felix. Bella was blind, her hearing was poor and her memory was markedly impaired, yet Felix found great purpose in caring for her and she found great meaning in being there for him. Gawande (2015: p. 56) writes:

> The physical presence of each other gave them comfort. He dressed her, bathed her, helped feed her. When they walked, they held hands. At night they lay in bed in each other's arms, awake and nestling for a while, before finally drifting off to sleep. Those moments, Felix said, remained among their most cherished. He felt they knew each other, and loved each other, more than at any time in their nearly seventy years together.

Here, we are reminded of how we began: the love between a mother and her baby that is nurtured through skin-to-skin contact is mirrored in the hidden physical intimacy of an older couple as they lay in each other's arms. Love and care may be expressed through simple physical closeness at any stage of life, from the very beginning to the very end.

References

Age UK (n.d.) Sex in later life. Available from: www.ageuk.org.uk/information-advice/health-wellbeing/relationships-family/sex-in-later-life/ (site accessed 24/11/2020).

Bramley, P. (ed.) (2009). *Doing anything after work ... what about retirement?* Great Hucklow: Hucklow Publishing.

Gawande, A. (2015) *Being mortal*. London: Wellcome Collection.

National Institute on Aging (n.d.) Sexuality in later life. Available from: www.nia.nih.gov/health/sexuality-later-life (site accessed 24/11/2020).

Further reading

Mayo Clinic (n.d.) Sexual health and aging: keep the passion alive. Available from: www.mayoclinic.org/healthy-lifestyle/sexual-health/in-depth/sexual-health/art-20046698 (site accessed 24/11/2020).

13 Supervision

Clinical supervision is essential for psychotherapy practice and in many other contexts, including health and social care. Addressing a succession of complex, sensitive issues can have a negative impact on any HP and consequently affect the quality of care they are able to provide. Clinical supervision is not HP therapy but rather a means to avoid any disruptions or blocks to the provision of high-quality care. Butterworth and Faugier (cited in Wells, 2000: p. 117) suggest that all practitioners – from senior staff to students – should set aside sufficient time to focus on the process and experience of the care they provide. The professional body for counsellors and psychotherapists – the British Association for Counselling and Psychotherapy – outlines the importance of clinical supervision for its members as follows: 'Clinical Supervision is a specialised form of mentoring provided for practitioners responsible for undertaking challenging work with people. Supervision is provided to ensure standards, enhance quality, advance learning, stimulate creativity and resilience of the work being undertaken' (BACP, n.d.).

Psychosexual therapy supervision should aim to address any unspoken reactions within the often complex therapist–patient relationship. Our skills require adaptation when addressing a human condition rather than a physical illness. The therapist is not 'the expert' nor there to 'make it better' (see Figures 0.1 and 0.2 in the Introduction); rather, their role is to consider the context of the presented problem, any potential links between that problem and physical symptoms, and the interconnections between mind, body and emotion.

In the absence of supervision, the therapist may respond on the basis of their own experiences, which can be detrimental to both their judgement and their skills. This can manifest as colluding with the patient, or developing maternal/paternal feelings towards them, either of which may block progress towards recovery. Even simply liking or disliking a patient on first meeting may prove problematic. During supervision it is essential not to judge these feelings but rather identify and explore the subconscious responses between therapist and patient.

It is imperative that the practitioner both feels safe and is completely honest with their supervisor. The supervisor should voice their concerns immediately if they believe that either of these elements is missing, and the contract should be terminated and alternative arrangements made if no solution can be found. It is also important to consider other concurrent relationships prior to selecting a supervisor. For example, it may be inappropriate for a therapist's line manager to act as their supervisor as such an arrangement may discourage total honesty. By contrast, peer supervision within agreed boundaries can aid learning as it provides unparalleled access to other practitioners' cases and experience.

Supervision should be used to reflect on what is going well along with any difficulties that may arise during therapy sessions. The added value of the process is that certain aspects of the therapy that the therapist had failed to notice may be identified. In addition, given the increasing complexity of publicly funded services, supervision helps therapists to recognise any gaps in their learning or training and provides information on where they may find the support they need.

As stated earlier, supervision is not 'counselling' for the therapist. Rather, it allows time for reflection on the cases themselves as well as the therapist's reactions, so it creates opportunities to identify prejudices and judgements that are based on personal life experience. This can be beneficial if it leads to conscious awareness of personal bias, but potentially detrimental if this is not recognised. It is important to acknowledge that assumptions based on personal experience may be at odds with the reality of the patient's experience.

Certain people and situations will always resonate with the therapist's personal experience more deeply than others; after all, every therapist is a human being, too. Equally, the patient may unconsciously transfer their feelings onto a particular HP who triggers memories of a significant experience.

Supervision cases

In this section, we revisit three cases in which supervision proved especially beneficial.

> **LOVELY LEONARD (SEE CHAPTER 5)**
>
> The therapist looked at her list for the day and said, 'Oh good, lovely Leonard …'
>
> Her colleague and peer supervisor replied, 'I think we had better discuss "Lovely Leonard" at our next supervision meeting.'
>
> During the subsequent meeting with her peer supervisor, the therapist's maternal feelings towards Leonard became more obvious to her. However, rather than these motherly feelings suffocating and stifling Leonard (see Figure 0.2 in the Introduction), it became clear through the case discussion that the therapist's holding relationship with him was actually supporting his growing self-awareness and increasing his confidence to make his own body, mind and emotional connections.
>
> The therapist took the reflections and insights she had gained during supervision back to her next session with Leonard and asked him directly if he felt she was being too motherly towards him. Leonard considered this question for some time before replying that he had not thought of her concern as maternal. This confirmed to the therapist the strong feeling in the room of Leonard as a lonely 12-year-old boy – a feeling of which he himself was unaware. By actively sharing with Leonard the observations that had emerged during her case supervision session, the therapist clarified for both of them that the intervention was helping Leonard to find his adult confidence.
>
> It can be difficult to avoid forming attachments to certain patients and feeling protective towards them, especially in long-term therapy. This is why it is essential to explore the relationship between patient and therapist at regular intervals. However, as we saw with Leonard, a healthy attachment may be beneficial in facilitating emotional growth and confidence.

Patients sometimes ask their therapists for personal information. Such requests should be considered very carefully, as acceding to them may lead the patient to make assumptions about the therapist and divert them from their own experiences. If a therapist does decide to share a few personal details, reflection during supervision will help to clarify whether this was an appropriate course of action.

We know of one therapist who was asked for details of her qualifications and experience. She proceeded to list all of her academic and practical qualifications and only then thought to ask the patient why she wanted to know. The patient seemed to have lost interest and replied, 'I just wanted to know if it was worth asking you to have a look at my rash!'

Every therapist will occasionally hear something that they find shocking or upsetting during therapy. In such circumstances, it is important not only to contain these feelings throughout the remainder of the session but also to share them during supervision. This is because, if left unaddressed, strong emotions can develop into what is known as 'vicarious trauma' and maybe even 'professional burnout' (Rothschild, 2006).

PRECIOUS' TIME (SEE CHAPTER 7)

Having faced a distraught patient falling to the floor and tearing at her clothes, the SHA later reflected that she had felt overwhelmed, so she raised the case at her next supervision meeting. This safe environment gave her the opportunity she needed to explore why the experience had been so distressing. She had delivered many positive HIV results in the past, but had never previously witnessed such a profound physical reaction.

'I had no idea what to do,' she admitted to her colleague. 'What could I do? Take her blood pressure? Get her some water? I couldn't get near enough to do either.'

Instead, she had simply remained quiet and sat on the floor next to Precious. After what had felt like an age, Precious had finally managed to express what she needed.

Nevertheless, in the safe space of supervision, the SHA was able to admit, 'But really all I wanted to do was run away!'

Within supervision, it is helpful to identify when a therapist is continuing with a patient for longer than is necessary, because this is often an indication of dependency. Many individuals are attracted to the caring professions in the hope of increasing their understanding of their own challenging experiences and to give others the help they feel they lacked. However, although this can be beneficial, it can also undermine the quality of care. For example, if meeting their own need for recognition remains a therapist's top priority, this will have a negative impact on their professional/therapeutic relationships. Moreover, becoming a patient's friend is likely to cloud the therapist's judgement and change the dynamic of the therapeutic engagement. Therefore, professional boundaries should be set and maintained to increase autonomy and reduce the risk of dependency.

Whenever a therapist meets a patient whom they know in some other capacity, it is essential to be transparent regarding the relationship and to check that the patient is happy to proceed. Support and reflection should be provided during supervision.

Supervision can also facilitate a therapist's withdrawal from any course of therapy in which they feel unsafe or manipulated by the patient. Such feelings should be reflected upon and considered carefully at one or more supervision meetings to support continued safe practice. We have all experienced unease when working with a particular patient and have utilised supervision to reach an objective decision regarding the best course of action for all concerned.

PEEPING TOM (SEE CHAPTER 6)

Due to Peeping Tom's presenting issue, the therapist decided to wear trousers whenever she was scheduled to see him. However, on one occasion, she arrived at work in a short dress, having forgotten she had an appointment with him that day. Although slightly worried when she saw his name on her list, she felt there was nothing she could do about it. As she reflected on the ensuing session during supervision, the therapist remarked that it had been unusually honest and challenging, even though she had been concerned that she might trigger a paraphilic response from Tom. Her supervisor responded, 'Maybe that was because you were being yourself, rather than trying to cover up. Being too careful can inhibit the work.' She then suggested reflecting with Tom that they had made considerable progress in their last session, despite her concerns about her attire. The therapist did just that, then asked Tom how he viewed her in respect to his paraphilia. He replied that it was not an issue for him because she was a professional woman to whom he could speak freely. With this boundary defined, the therapist felt free to wear whatever she liked.

As HPs, we need to be aware that we can make unconscious judgements about any of our patients. These may be recognised and addressed during supervision, such as when supervisors spotted one therapist's maternal feelings for Leonard and another's identification of Tom as a potential threat. Exploring such issues in clinical supervision can transform them from problems into sources of learning and enhanced practice.

Maintaining professional boundaries during therapy

Discussing boundaries at the start of a course of therapy and drafting a contract help to ensure a safe working environment for both parties. The contract that is agreed during the first session should always stipulate that either party retains the right to end the therapy at any time. Moreover, if there has been a previous professional or personal relationship between patient and therapist, this should be explored to establish whether a therapeutic relationship is appropriate or advisable. It may prove difficult to resolve certain risks relating to the breaching of boundaries, in which case these should be addressed in clinical supervision in order to protect both the patient and the therapist. In rare cases, the therapist may still feel unsafe, for example if the patient is particularly aggressive or develops an inappropriate fixation. Such situations should be discussed at the earliest opportunity during supervision in order to determine the best way forward. If the decision is made to terminate the therapy, the patient should be advised on alternative sources of help.

Whilst it is important for patients to be completely honest during psychosexual therapy – for instance, they should be encouraged to disclose recreational drug use as well as sexual preferences and activity – boundaries must be re-enforced if any harmful behaviour comes to light. In addition, it might be necessary to terminate the therapy and inform the appropriate agencies. For example, if a patient discloses that they have acted on their sexual attraction to children, the relevant safeguarding procedures should be followed. Similarly, safeguarding actions will need to be implemented if a patient is considered at serious risk of self-harm or vulnerable to attacks by others. This is why it is important to discuss confidentiality boundaries at the start of every course of therapy and include any circumstances when they may be breached in the contract.

A patient will often re-experience buried feelings during therapy. If these are transferred onto and felt towards the therapist, this is known as 'transference'. A degree of transference is to be expected within the therapeutic relationship; indeed, it may even prove useful. However, there are times when it – or 'counter-transference', in which the roles are reversed and the therapist transfers feelings onto the patient – is both inappropriate and destructive. Counter-transference is more complex than transference because the therapist is often unaware of the emotions that have been triggered by their relationship with the patient (Skrine, 1997: p. 29). This is illustrated in the following case study.

ARIEL'S ANNOYANCE

Ariel, who was born male, started short-term psychosexual therapy at the age of 23 to explore their gender identity as a trans female. They had been struggling to fit in as far back as they could remember and were full of anger because they attributed their ongoing confusion to others' mistakes. Ariel was still in a heterosexual relationship with Dayna, who had been questioning her own gender identity long before Ariel had started to do the same. Ariel was desperate to understand their own years of chaotic relationships, brief connections and painful disruptions. They insisted they had tried to cause as little disruption as possible at work following their name change, but relationships with colleagues had deteriorated rapidly and they were subsequently dismissed. As a result, they were now taking legal action against their employer for unfair dismissal.

THE THERAPIST'S REFLECTION

The therapist became increasingly confused, exasperated and irritated with Ariel as they immediately dismissed every suggestion for moving forward. Although the therapist was able to acknowledge that this was a problematic reaction, she felt exhausted and started dreading their sessions, not least because Ariel continued to blame others for their distress.

Exploration of the therapeutic relationship during supervision largely focused on the therapist's irritability and concerns that she too would soon face an official complaint. The supervisor and therapist both felt that Ariel had made little or no progress in accepting personal responsibility for their issues, and suspected that they would probably change direction once again in their search for a secure identity.

The supervisor questioned the suitability of the therapy and wondered whether it might be triggering something from the therapist's past. She suggested that the therapist might have transferred her frustration onto Ariel, leading to mutual irritability and feelings of failure. The therapist shared these ideas during her next session with Ariel and asked if they thought the supervisor was correct. Once the situation had been acknowledged and both parties had agreed that they were making no progress, they decided to conclude the therapy and Ariel was put in touch with gender identity support groups. Much to the therapist's surprise, on the client feedback form, Ariel not only expressed their gratitude for the therapy but rated it highly.

REFLECT

For Ariel, the therapeutic relationship may have mirrored their relationships with others and indeed themself. Aspects of the autistic spectrum, Borderline Personality Disorder and narcissism were all noted during the sessions and appeared to contribute to Ariel's struggle to develop an acceptable identity. As illustrated, clinical supervision helps to negate the risk of counter-transference becoming a block to effective care.

RESPOND

This case led the therapist to a deeper understanding of the lived experiences of individuals who need, at minimum, full acknowledgement and appreciation of their specific context and personal identity. It also revealed the complexity of motivations, including emotional responses to frustration and the profound desire to find a personal identity that not only fits internally but also enables better social engagement. Finally, it is important to recognise when the therapy process has stalled and to share this with the patient in order to identify the best way forward, even if this entails ending therapy.

Peer supervision and further support

As well as regular, contracted clinical supervision, health and social care professionals may utilise peer supervision and further support. Peer supervision, which is usually less formal than clinical supervision, provides a safe, non-judgemental space for confidential discussions with one or more trusted colleagues in the interests of developing insights and enhancing learning. This can be just as effective as other, more structured forms of learning and team-building.

Similarly, self-care supports effective practice when working with people who are facing complex life challenges. It is crucial to maintain a balance among activities, projects, hobbies, relationships, good nutrition, rest and exercise, along with professional training and development (BACP, 2018). Commissioners of services, employers, teams and colleagues in the caring professions all have a responsibility to ensure that supervision and self-care remain integral parts of a healthy and effective professional life to support the safe delivery of services.

Professional training and support

In the UK, the College of Sexual and Relationship Therapists (COSRT, n.d.) provides validated specialist training in psychosexual and relationship therapy. In addition, the Institute of Psychosexual Medicine now offers validated training for doctors and other health professionals who routinely conduct intimate physical examinations as part of their clinical role (IPM, n.d.).

A number of UK charities, including RELATE, also offer training in sexual and relationship therapy (RELATE, n.d.), while various professional organisations provide short courses to assist continued professional development. Full details are available through the organisations' websites or from experts in the field.

To maintain competence, every HP should continue to undertake clinical supervision, professional education and training throughout their working life.

References

BACP (2018). Self-care for the counselling professions. Available from: www.bacp.co.uk/media/3939/bacp-self-care-fact-sheet-gpia088-jul18.pdf (site accessed 24/11/2020).

BACP (n.d.). Ethical framework. Available from: www.bacp.co.uk/events-and-resources/ethics-and-standards/ethical-framework-for-the-counselling-professions/supervision/ (site accessed 06/020/2021).

COSRT (n.d.) Training and validation for HPs and couple therapists in psychosexual therapy. Available from: www.cosrt.org.uk/(site accessed 24/11/2020).

IPM (n.d.). Institute of Psychosexual Medicine (IPM). Available from: www.rcog.org.uk/en/about-us/specialist-societies/institute-of-psychosexual-medicine-ipm/ (site accessed 24/11/2020).

RELATE (n.d.) RELATE Professional Certificate in Psychosexual Therapy. Available from: www.relate.org.uk/about-us/work-us/train-be-counsellor/relate-professional-certificate-psychosexual-therapy/ (site accessed 24/11/2020).
Rothschild, B. (2006) *Help for the helper: the psychophysiology of compassion fatigue and vicarious trauma*. New York: Norton.
Skrine, R. (1997) *Blocks and freedoms in sexual life*. Oxford: Radcliffe.
Wells, D. (ed.) (2000) *Caring for sexuality in health and illness*. London: Churchill Livingstone.

Further reading

Counselling Resource (n.d.) Counselling and therapy supervision. Available from: https://counsellingresource.com/therapy/aboutcouns/supervision/ (site accessed 24/11/2020).

UK professional bodies

- Balint Society UK (Registered Charity 261387): https://balint.co.uk/about/the-balint-method/
- British Association for Counselling and Psychotherapy (BACP): www.bacp.co.uk
- British Association for Sexual Health and HIV (BASHH): www.bashh.org
- College of Sexual and Relationship Therapy (COSRT): www.cosrt.org.uk
- Community Practitioners and Health Visitors Association (CPHVA): https://maternalmentalhealthalliance.org/member/community-practitioners-and-health-visitors-association-cphva/
- Institute of Health Visiting: https://ihv.org.uk
- Institute of Psychosexual Medicine (IPM): www.ipm.org.uk
- Nursing and Midwifery Council (NMC): www.nmc.org.uk
- Royal College of Midwives (RCM): www.rcm.org.uk
- Royal College of Obstetricians and Gynaecologists (RCOG): www.rcog.org.uk
- Society of Sexual Health Advisors (SSHA): https://ssha.info/resources/i-want-to-be-a-health-adviser/

Epilogue

We have known each other professionally in various clinical settings, but our true connection was developed through the Association of Psychosexual Nursing and especially its biannual national seminars in Soho, London. The latter involved an early Saturday morning trip to London, a day of seminars, speakers and reflection, and usually the brief treat of some shopping. A takeaway glass of wine and some snacks would fuel lots of chatter on the train journey home, even as we attempted to lower our volume when words such as 'sex', 'arousal', 'erectile dysfunction' and 'vaginismus' slipped out!

It was during one of these intense conversations that we acknowledged the full importance and potential of psychosexual therapy in so many circumstances. We reflected on countless examples of simple but skilled interventions and the positive outcomes that may be achieved when we have the courage to address physical intimacy. For instance, we recalled the story of a palliative care nurse who had been bold enough to ask a couple if they had considered their sexual relationship, despite a recent terminal diagnosis. This opened the door to a heartfelt expression of the couple's deep grief and consequent recognition that they could still enjoy a meaningful physical connection. Following this candid discussion, they were able to rediscover their physical intimacy, which was a great comfort to both of them.

As the three of us discussed all of the professional contexts in which we had used our psychosexual skills we started to appreciate the true value of those skills and wondered how we might share our wealth of experience. Judy suggested that we should record our experiences and at that moment we embarked on the journey that led to this book.

There were several pauses along the way, but on reflection these were highly beneficial, as they allowed us to reassess and update the book with further examples of intimacy, sex and relationship challenges.

We remain passionate about this subject and hope that our enthusiasm, experience and insights will serve to motivate others. We wrote this book in a novel way – working together rather than independently – which resulted in more than a few heated debates about certain words and phrases. Nevertheless, after countless cups of coffee, sunshine, showers, some tears and a great deal of laughing at ourselves, we emerged with our friendship and mutual respect not only intact but enriched. Through this process we have recognised, shared and accepted our own vulnerabilities, as you have seen mirrored in our work.

Covid-19

This book was completed during the Covid-19 pandemic, which gave us some unexpected extra time to focus and reflect on the content. On the other hand, the physical restrictions associated with the crisis meant that connection with one another was suddenly limited, and we were denied much of the intimacy and closeness that the majority of human beings crave. Like most other people in the UK, we have had to resort to virtual alternatives to meet those needs.

As we write, the hidden anger, uncertainty and sense of powerlessness that the pandemic has engendered are still disrupting personal relationships and family life across the generations. Some may have welcomed the reduced social interaction of lockdown, but the restrictions have been unbearable for many. As therapists, our main concern is how the lack of physical and emotional contact will impact on social and sexual relationships and wellbeing in the future. The pandemic has raised concerns about deteriorating mental and physical health, domestic violence, lost earnings and suicide. Our aim, both professionally and personally, is to develop the skills and confidence in others to address intimacy, sex and relationship challenges effectively maximising physical and mental health.

Judy, Sue and Jean

Index

Intimacy, Sex and Relationship Challenges: Index.
Locators in *italics* refer to figures.

abortion 44–46, 53–54
abuse *see* childhood sexual abuse (CSA)
adolescence: case study 21–22; disabilities 58; gender reassignment services 16; influences on sexual development 21; teenage pregnancy 36–39
ageing *see* mid-life; older age
andropause 132–135
anxiety 67–69
arousal: and desire 78–79, 82–84; differences in expectation 82–84; fetishes 88–89; sexual function/dysfunction 12
arranged marriages 115, 120–121
Asexual Visibility & Education Network (AVEN) 11
asexuality 76–77, 92
assisted reproduction 48–49, 123
Association of Psychosexual Nursing 161
Autistic Spectrum Disorder (ASD) 14, 69–72

babies *see* infants
Balint, Enid 2
Balint, Michael 2
bereavement 124–126, 141–142, 146–147
biological sex: gender identity 14–15; intersex 15; sexual attraction 11

bisexual attraction 11
British Association for Counselling and Psychotherapy 150

cancer diagnoses 136–138
cervical smear test 108–110
child development: disabilities 58–60, 62–63; disruption to sexual development 22–24; first relationships and early sexual development 20; influences on sexual development 21
child sexual exploitation (CSE) 27–31
childbirth 50–52
childhood sexual abuse (CSA) 24–27, 103–107
chlamydia 85–86
civil partnerships 114–118
clinical supervision 150–155
College of Sexual and Relationship Therapists (COSRT) 158
colposcopy 110–113
confidentiality 155
consensual nonmonogamy 85–88
continuing professional development: clinical supervision 150–155; peer supervision 157–158; Reflect and Respond model (R&R) 6–7
counter-transference 155–156
Covid-19 pandemic 162
cross-dressing 81

164 Index

depression 67–69, 92
desire: and arousal 78–79, 82–84; asexuality 11; case study 22–23; differences in 73, 78–84; impact of sexual abuse 103–104; infertility 48–49; menopause 129; mid-life 127–129; polyamory 87–88; sexual function/dysfunction 12; termination of pregnancy 45–46; traumatic experiences 54–55
Diagnostic Statistical Manual of Mental Disorders (DSM-5) 13–14
disabled people: acquired physical disability 60–62; learning-disabled challenges 62–64; physical and mental challenges 58–60; physically and mentally disabled babies 57–58
drug trafficking 28

early years: child sexual exploitation (CSE) 27–31; childhood sexual abuse (CSA) 24–27; disruption to sexual development 22–24; female genital mutilation (FGM) 31–34; first relationships and early sexual development 20; influences on sexual development 21
emotions: as cause of sexual dysfunction 9; child sexual exploitation 29; childhood sexual abuse 26–27; clinical supervision 152–153; disruption to sexual development 22–24; loss of full health 141; postnatal 123–124; pregnancy 41; sexual health 94–95; surgery and medical conditions 136–138; termination of pregnancy 45–46; traumatic experiences 52–55
erectile dysfunction: arousal 83–84; infertility 47–48; in marriage 115; mid-life 134–135; new relationships 122, 124
exhibitionism 88

female genital mutilation (FGM) 31–34
fertility: contraceptive provision 39–41; in-vitro fertilisation (IVF) 48–49, 123; infertility 47–48; menopause 128–129; pregnancy 41–44; teenage pregnancy 36–39

fetishes 88–91
frotteurism 88

gays *see* homosexuality
gender dysphoria 13–14
gender identity: biological sex 14–15; exploration of 73–78, 156; incongruence 16–17; *see also* transgender
gender identity disorder 13–14
gender reassignment services 16–17
genderqueer 77; *see also* non-binary
genital examination *see* intimate physical examination
grooming 27–31

health professional (HP): childhood sexual abuse 25–26; female genital mutilation 32–33, 34; meaning of term xiv; Reflect and Respond model (R&R) 2, 4–6; sexual health 95–97; teenage pregnancy 38; *see also* therapeutic relationship
heart attack 139–141
homosexuality: civil partnership 114, 118; exploration of 79–81; polyamory 85–86; sexual desire case study 22–23
'hot flushes' 130–131
Human Immunodeficiency Virus (HIV) 97, 100–103
human rights, female genital mutilation 32
hymen 115
hysteroscopy 110–113

in-vitro fertilisation (IVF) 48–49, 123
infants: mother-and-baby relationship 20; postnatal emotions 123–124; *see also* early years
infertility 47–48; in-vitro fertilisation (IVF) 48–49, 123; menopause 128–129
Institute of Psychosexual Medicine (IPM) 2–3
International Classification of Diseases (ICD) 13–14
intersex 15; *see also* transgender
intimacy: across the lifespan xiii–xv; discussion in healthcare setting 1; expectations about 10

intimate physical examination: cervical smear test 108–110; colposcopy and hysteroscopy 110–113; STI screening 97–98; women's health 108

labour (childbirth) 50–52
learning-disabled challenges 62–64
life expectancy 127
loss of full health 138–142
loss of sexual pleasure 120–126
losses in reproductive years: disruption of childbirth 50–52; infertility 47–48; miscarriage 48–50; near-death experiences and stillbirth 52–55; Sudden Infant Death Syndrome (SIDS) 23, 125; termination of pregnancy 44–46

male menopause 132
marriage 114–118
mastectomy 136
masturbation 23
media, influences on sexual development 21
medical diagnoses, mid-life 135–138
medically unexplained symptoms (MUS) 7–8
menopause 128–132
menstruation 128
mental health: anxiety and depression 67–69; Autistic Spectrum Disorder (ASD) 14, 69–72; depression 92; gender reassignment services 17; impact on sexual function 65; Obsessive Compulsive Disorder (OCD) 65–67, 71; transgender communities 16
mid-life 127–128; andropause 132–135; losses and gains 138–142; menopause 128–132; surgery and medical conditions 135–138
miscarriage 48–50
mother-and-baby relationship 20

near-death experiences, childbirth 52–55
non-binary 15, 76–78

Obsessive Compulsive Disorder (OCD) 65–67, 71

older age: adapting to 144–145; new challenges 146–148; realities of sexual activity 148–149
oral sexual assault 104
orgasm 10, 12

paedophilia 88, 155
pain: first-time having sex 114–117; menopause 130–131; during sex 49–50; sexual dysfunction 12; therapy for 110; umbilical cord prolapse 51–52
paraphilia 88–91, 154
'partner swapping' 85
Patient Health Questionnaire Somatic Symptom Severity (PHQ-15) 24–27
peer supervision 157–158
physical closeness 147, 149
physical disability: acquired 60–62; from birth 57–58; physical and mental challenges 58–60
physical examination *see* intimate physical examination
polyamory 85–88
pornography 23–24
postnatal emotions 123–124
practitioner–patient relationship *see* therapeutic relationship
pre-exposure prophylaxis (PrEP) 100
pregnancy: in adolescence 36–39; case studies 42–44; childbirth 50–52; emotional response 41; infertility 47–48; termination 44–46
premature ejaculation (PE) 115
privacy 128
professional boundaries 154, 155–158
professional development: clinical supervision 150–155; peer supervision 157–158; Reflect and Respond model (R&R) 6–7
professional training 158
psychoanalytic perspectives 2–3
psychosexual awareness 2–3
puberty-blockers 16

rapid ejaculation (RE) 115, 122
Reflect and Respond model (R&R) 2; adolescent case study 21–22; andropause 133–134; arousal 83, 84; asexuality 92; bereavement 124–126;

166 Index

child sexual exploitation 29–30, 31; childbirth 51, 52; childhood sexual abuse 26, 27; contraceptive provision 41; disabilities 58, 59, 60, 62, 63, 64; disruption to sexual development 24; female genital mutilation 34; infertility 48; intimate physical examination 109–110; marriage and civil partnerships 115–116, 117, 118; menopause 131–132; mental health 66–69, 70, 72; miscarriage 50; older age 145–148; paraphilia 89–90, 91; polyamory 86, 87–88; pregnancy 42, 43, 44; process template 6–7, *7*; sexual assault 105–107; sexual health 96, 97, 98–100, 101–103; sexual health services 40; sexuality 80–82; teenage pregnancy 37, 38–39; therapeutic relationship 4–6, 157; transgender 74–75, 77, 78; traumatic experiences 54, 55
reflective practice 4–5
relationship therapy training (RELATE) 158
reproductive years: contraceptive provision 39–41; infertility 47–48; pregnancy 41–44; teenage pregnancy 36–39; termination of pregnancy 44–46; *see also* losses in reproductive years
retirement 148–149; *see also* older age

sado-masochism 88
safeguarding 25, 155
same-sex attraction 11
same-sex relationships: civil partnership 114, 118; exploration of 79–81; polyamory 85–86; sexual desire case study 22–23
sex: first-time 114–117, 118; motivations for 11, *12*; pressures on adolescents 21
sex and relationship education (SRE) 36
sex chromosomes 15
sexual abuse 24–27, 103–107
sexual assault 103
sexual attraction: asexuality 11; disabilities 61–62; and motivation 11; *see also* desire

sexual development: disabilities 57–64; first relationships and early sexual development 20; influences on 21
sexual expressions 10
sexual fetishes 88
sexual function/dysfunction: across the lifespan xiii–xv; causes of dysfunction 7–10, *8*; defining dysfunction 11–14; discussion in healthcare setting 1; expert's role in discussion *3*, 3–4; infertility 47–48; loss of pleasure 120–126; marriage and civil partnerships 114–118; mental health 65
sexual health: across the lifespan 94; consultation 95–97; Human Immunodeficiency Virus (HIV) 97, 100–103; therapeutic relationship 94–95; unexpected disclosures of sexual abuse and assault 103–107
sexual health services 39–41
sexual history 30, 94
sexual pleasure, loss of 120–126
sexuality: expectations about 10; exploration of 79–81; mid-life 134; transgender 73–78
sexually transmitted infections (STIs): chlamydia 85–86; clinical discussion 94–95; older age 147; risk of contracting 95, 97–98; screening 97–100
smear test 108–110
sport, and gender identity 15
stillbirth 52–55
Sudden Infant Death Syndrome (SIDS) 23, 125
suicide, gender incongruence 16
supervision, clinical 150–155
surgery 135–138
swab tests 97–98
'swinging' 85

termination of pregnancy 44–46; *see also* losses in reproductive years
testosterone: andropause 132; gender identity 15
therapeutic relationship: clinical supervision 150–155; expert's role in discussion *3*, 3–4; peer supervision 157–158; professional boundaries 154, 155–158; professional contexts

161–162; Reflect and Respond model (R&R) 2, 4–6; training and applied principles 2–3
therapeutic space 6
therapy process 9
transference 155–156, 157
transgender: cross-dressing 81; definition 73; exploration of 73–78, 156; gender incongruence 16; non-binary 15; suicide rates 16
traumatic experiences: child sexual exploitation (CSE) 27–31; childbirth 50–52; childhood sexual abuse (CSA) 24–27, 103–107; near-death experiences and stillbirth 52–55; surgery and medical conditions 136–137

United Nations Convention on the Rights of the Child 32

unresolved persistent physical symptoms (uPPS): causes of sexual dysfunction 8–10, 9; childhood sexual abuse 26–27; as cycle 25
urine tests 97–98

vaginal dryness 129
vaginal ring pessary 144
vaginismus 109, 116–117, 120, 145
Valins, L. 10
Viagra 148
voyeurism 88, 90–91

widowhood 141–142, 146
women's health: cervical smear test 108–110; colposcopy and hysteroscopy 110–113; intimate physical examination 108; menopause 128–132; *see also* reproductive years

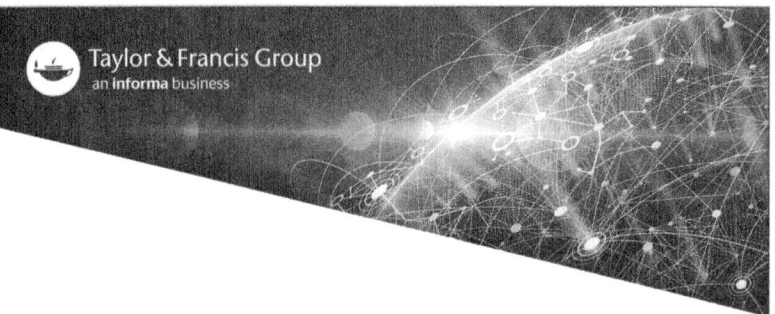